Obstetrical Intervention and Technology in the 1980s

D1528036

ABOUT THE EDITOR

Diony Young is an educator, consultant and advocate in maternal and child health. She is the author of *Changing Childbirth: Family Birth in the Hospital*, 1982.

Ms. Young is a consultant to the International Childbirth Education Association and has served on the Board of Directors of that organization and the Finger Lakes Health Systems Agency. She is also on the Advisory Committee on Accreditation and Curriculum Development of the American College of Nurse-Midwives and participated in the Governor's Conference for the Prevention of Developmental Disabilities and Infant Mortality in New York.

Obstetrical Intervention and Technology in the 1980s

Diony Young, Editor

Women & Health
Volume 7, Numbers 3/4

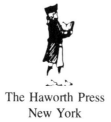

The Haworth Press
New York

RG
541
027
1983

The Haworth Press, Inc., 28 East 22 Street, New York, NY 10010.

Library of Congress Cataloging in Publication Data
Main entry under title:

Obstetrical intervention and technology in the 1980s.

    (Women & health ; v. 7, no. 3/4)
    Includes bibliographical references.
    1. Obstetrics—Addresses, essays, lectures. I. Young, Diony, 1938- . II. Series. [DNLM:
1. Obstetrics—Trends. W1 W0478 v. 7 no. 3/4 / WQ 100 01346]
RG541.027 1983   618.2   82-21301
ISBN 0-86656-143-9

Obstetrical Intervention and Technology in the 1980s

Women & Health
Volume 7, Numbers 3/4

Contents

CONTRIBUTORS

H. David Banta, MD, MPH
Health Program Manager
Office of Technology Assessment
Washington, D.C.

Christopher L. Christman, PhD
Senior Research Engineer, Acoustic
    Radiation Branch
Division of Biological Effects
Bureau of Radiological Health
Food and Drug Administration
Rockville, Maryland

Paul L. Doering, MS
Associate Professor of Pharmacy Practice
Director, Drug Information and Pharmacy
    Resource Center
College of Pharmacy
University of Florida
Gainesville, Florida

Samuel Gorovitz, PhD
Professor and Chairman
Department of Philosophy
University of Maryland
College Park, Maryland

David Graham, MD, FRCS (C)
Assistant Professor, Obstetrics and
    Gynecology
Assistant Professor, Radiology
The Johns Hopkins Medical Institutions
Baltimore, Maryland

Albert D. Haverkamp, MD, FACOG
Director of Perinatal Research
Obstetrical and Gynecological Departments
Denver General Hospital and University of
    Colorado Medical School
Denver, Colorado

Brigitte Jordan, PhD
Associate Professor of Anthropology and
    Pediatrics
Department of Anthropology
College of Osteopathic Medicine
Michigan State University
East Lansing, Michigan

Irwin H. Kaiser, MD, PhD
Professor
Department of Gynecology and Obstetrics
Albert Einstein College of Medicine of
    Yeshiva University
Bronx Municipal Hospital Center
The Bronx, New York

Judith Lumley, MA, MBBS, PhD
Senior Lecturer
Department of Obstetrics and Gynecology
Monash University
Queen Victoria Medical Centre
Melbourne, Australia

Helen I. Marieskind, DrPH
Executive Director
Vision Services, An Agency for the
    Visually Impaired
Seattle, Washington

Miriam Orleans, PhD
Professor
Department of Preventive Medicine
University of Colorado Health Sciences
    Center
Denver, Colorado

Penelope P. Simkin, RPT
Childbirth Educator and Lecturer
Seattle, Washington

Melvin E. Stratmeyer, PhD
Chief, Acoustic Radiation Branch
Division of Biological Effects
Bureau of Radiological Health
Food and Drug Administration
Rockville, Maryland

Stephen B. Thacker, MD
Chief, Consolidated Surveillance and
    Communications Activity
Centers for Disease Control
Atlanta, Georgia

Special Contribution

Committee of Technical Bulletins
of The American College of Obstetricians and Gynecologists
The American College of Obstetricians and Gynecologists
Washington, D.C.

PREFACE

Obstetrics in the 1970s has embraced the era of medical technology with enthusiasm. The developing technologies of ultrasound and amniocentesis, and the surgical management of birth have together transformed childbearing into a medical and surgical model of care. Their medical, social, and economic impact on birth and family outcome continues to be assessed. As we move into the 1980s, it is apparent that these technologies more and more will become an accepted part of obstetrical care. Of major concern is the fact that the rapid advances in technology are frequently outstripping medical knowledge about them and their ultimate effect on human health.

The purpose of this monograph, *Obstetrical Intervention and Technology in the 1980s*, is to examine some of the technologies used in obstetrics today and describe the current state of knowledge about them. It is the first monograph in a series that will address different issues in women's health care, planned for publication by *Women & Health*.

Technology in obstetrics has an important place. The issue of its *rightful* place in pregnancy, labor, and birth management is one of never-ending controversy, as many of the contributors in this monograph point out. One of the great concerns is that so many of the interventive practices carried out routinely in many hospitals today have never been demonstrated in properly controlled, scientific investigations to benefit healthy women and babies. As the argument is voiced that pregnancy itself is a pathological condition requiring the ultimate in high-risk management, the realization that women can no longer labor and give birth without medical and surgical assistance is beginning to come true. Indeed, the expectation of complications becomes self-fulfilling, as different interventions and technologies take their psychological and physiological effect.

The extraordinarily thorny ethical and moral issues involved in the emergence and increasing sophistication of obstetrical technology have been examined by Samuel Gorovitz in the introduction of this monograph. He emphasizes that sensitivity to, and understanding of, the conflicts of values inevitable in an expanding medical care technology are not enough—a purposeful effort must be made by care providers to deal with them.

Antepartum fetal heart rate testing has attained an increasing role in antenatal care. Judith Lumley has examined the safety, reliability, and con-

xi

tribution to a better outcome of these tests, which include the oxytocin challenge tests, nonstress tests, and unstressed cardiotocography. One may also speculate on the possible future of the alternative or supplement to these tests—that of using the mother herself to monitor the movements of her fetus.

The second part of Judith Lumley's paper discusses the controversial subject of induction of labor. It has been suggested recently that a more liberal use of induction would decrease perinatal mortality. Lumley critically examines the justification for this view.

Irwin Kaiser, in the paper that follows, discusses the significant and expanding contribution of amniocentesis to investigating the status of the fetus. The uses of the procedure are described, but as Kaiser points out, these must be measured against its risks. In addition, amniocentesis presents difficult ethical and legal problems, which are considered in this paper.

Three papers follow on the diagnostic use of ultrasound, each one covering a different aspect of this technology. It was considered that the complexity of ultrasound, as well as its increasing impact on obstetrical management, warranted additional attention. The first paper, by David Graham, describes the current ways in which ultrasound is used in clinical obstetrical practice. This is followed by a previously published *ACOG Technical Bulletin*, entitled, "Diagnostic Ultrasound in Obstetrics and Gynecology," by The American College of Obstetricians and Gynecologists. In addition to methods and use of ultrasound, this paper addresses the subjects of safety, routine versus indicated use, and pitfalls in ultrasound diagnosis. The third paper in the group, by Melvin Stratmeyer and Christopher Christman, examines the biological effects of ultrasound. It describes the basic principles and mechanisms of action of this technology, followed by a review of human and laboratory studies that demonstrate the gaps in knowledge about ultrasound-induced bioeffects and, hence, the difficulty in assessing its safety.

External cephalic version, a procedure not commonly practiced in the United States, is presented by Brigitte Jordan. She discusses this procedure from the standpoint of offering a third alternative to the standard methods of breech delivery, which today is increasingly managed by cesarean section or vaginal delivery in selected cases. She traces the history and cross-cultural aspects of this procedure and then discusses its three approaches—the traditional approach, the conventional medical approach, and the more recent tocolytic version approach. The risks and benefits of version are assessed based on a comprehensive review of the literature.

Amniotomy, the surgical rupture of the membranes, is presented by Penelope Simkin. In reviewing the literature, she compares amniotomy with spontaneous rupture of the membranes and examines the procedure as a means both to induce and to augment labor. Based on the evidence, Simkin assesses the efficacy and appropriateness of this commonly practiced intervention.

Albert Haverkamp and Miriam Orleans provide a current assessment of electronic fetal monitoring. The almost universal use of this procedure in both uncomplicated and complicated obstetrical management has precipitated widespread controversy. Haverkamp and Orleans review the evidence for its efficacy, its impact on perinatal mortality, its effect on the cesarean section rate, and finally, offer some recommendations for its appropriate use.

Obstetrical analgesia and anesthesia, by Paul Doering, is intended to provide women and their partners with information that will allow them ''to be better decision makers about the obstetrical use of drugs.'' He describes both the action and safety of drugs on mother and fetus, based on a review of current literature. This paper is completed with a helpful discussion of patient rights and responsibilities concerning the use of drugs in labor and birth.

Stephen Thacker and David Banta provide a comprehensive discussion of the benefits and risks of episiotomy—a surgical procedure that is being increasingly questioned and the benefits of which, as the evidence clearly demonstrates, are lacking. The authors point out that the risks of episiotomy have been largely ignored, and it is essential for women to be able to make an informed decision about whether or not they will undergo this procedure. This paper provides the facts that will help them make that choice.

The final paper, by Helen Marieskind, discusses cesarean section, a major surgical procedure that has become commonplace in the management of birth as we enter the 1980s. The subject is given a historical perspective, followed by a description of the procedure, a discussion of complications, and possible explanations for the recent rise in the cesarean section rate. Cesarean section, like other obstetrical interventions, has an appropriate place in birth management, Marieskind observes, but careful evaluation of its application and benefits should have been performed before its widespread adoption.

Certain key concepts about obstetrical intervention and technology in the 1980s deserve additional emphasis.

First, essential to the proper use of technology is an acceptance of the woman's right to be informed about all aspects of a procedure or treatment and how it will affect her and her baby. This sharing of information will not only enable a woman to make decisions about her care appropriate to her special situation, but it will enhance the communications and relationship between her and her care providers. In this way birth outcome, parent outcome, and provider outcome will all benefit.

Second, the proper use of technology requires its integration with a family-centered philosophy and model of care. Thus the necessary emotional and social elements inherent in childbirth will add a vital and humanistic dimension to obstetrical care.

Third, the proper use of intervention and technology requires that they be used on a selective basis and that valid and proved indications be present before any procedure is applied to childbearing women. The routine use of obstetrical practices is no longer considered appropriate by many authorities for labor and birth management.

Finally, the clinical use of obstetrical interventions and technology must be preceded by scientifically valid studies and their results carefully evaluated before a practice is introduced into obstetrical care. Interventions and procedures in current use should come under critical scrutiny and be discarded if evidence of their benefits is absent.

The valuable contribution of technology to maternal and fetal well-being is indisputable. But that value is diminished unless technology is used with caution and applied only in situations of proven benefit.

The contributions of the authors who have shared their expertise in the writing of this monograph are acknowledged with gratitude by *Women & Health*. Their papers have drawn together in one publication an impressive body of thought-provoking knowledge on intervention and technology in obstetrics that will be an invaluable resource for both health professionals and health consumers in the future. That information, in turn, can be effectively utilized in clinical practice to improve the health and outcome of mothers and babies everywhere.

As Guest Editor, I wish to express my sincere gratitude to Dr. Helen Marieskind, Editor of *Women & Health*, and Dr. Irwin Kaiser for their thoughtful reviews of the papers in this monograph. Their valuable suggestions and encouragement have added substantially to the usefulness of this text.

Diony Young
Guest Editor

Obstetrical Intervention and Technology in the 1980s

INTRODUCTION:
THE ETHICAL ISSUES

Samuel Gorovitz

A woman gives birth to a grossly malformed infant who cannot live, but has not died. Modern technology makes it possible to sustain the life of the infant for an indeterminate period. The physician wonders: How vigorously, if at all, should we treat this child? Perhaps we should just let it die, or even hasten its death. What should I tell the mother in the meantime? Should I allow her to participate in these decisions, or would that be a shirking of my own responsibilities, imposing undue burdens on her at a time of great vulnerability? And why was I never taught anything in medical school to help me deal with situations like this?

A woman asks her physician for amniocentesis because the family has three sons, and she wants to terminate her pregnancy unless the child will be a girl. The physician wonders: Is this a misuse of medical technology? Is it up to me to pass judgment on the woman's reasons for wanting to know the sex of her fetus, or for wanting an abortion? Must I respect her request? Would it be right for me to do so? Is there anywhere I can turn for advice on how to deal with this dilemma?

A woman and her husband want a child of their own. But the woman does not want to be pregnant; it would interfere with her career. The couple have found another woman who is willing to have their embryo implanted in her uterus and to carry the fetus to term for them as a surrogate mother. They ask a physician to aid them in this plan by arranging *in vitro* fertilization. The physician wonders: Is this what I became a doctor for—to be a consulting engineer to help in the manufacture of children? Or am I just being an old fossil, having difficulty adjusting to the expanded range of choices made possible by scientific progress? Are these advances in medical technology a benefit to humankind, or are they steps in the direction of social decay? And amidst all these new possibilities, what ought I to do?

A pregnant woman confronts her gynecologist with the fact that although her first child was born by low transverse cesarean section, she intends to have her second child at home. She has been studying the literature on cesarean delivery and is well armed with statistics. She believes the evidence

1

demonstrates that the risk she runs by having a home birth, although real, is small, and she and her husband are strongly opposed to what they see as an unnatural reliance in medicine on high technology. The physician wonders: Should I just dismiss this woman on the grounds that if she doesn't do things my way, I won't be involved at all? She's been my patient for years, and I don't want just to abandon her. But I have failed completely to get her to change her mind. Can I *order* her to deliver in the hospital? Does she have the right to jeopardize her life and that of her child like this? Do I have an obligation to respect her decision and stand by her? Why can't I find a word about such problems in any of my medical books?

These vignettes are not science fiction. They do not involve flights of fancy about clones, chimeras, cryogenic miracles, or any other libertine extrapolations from present possibilities to a frightening future. They describe episodes that are real today and are more and more becoming a part of the fabric of everyday medical practice. Physicians, their patients, and the larger society are ill prepared to deal with them well.

Such problems are especially prominent in obstetrical practice, where birth and death, and our increasing ability to manipulate them, are central phenomena. That increasing ability results in large measure from the availability of new medical technologies, but it would be a mistake to think that technology is the source of the problems. Technology provides us with a wider array of choices than we have previously known; our moral anxiety in the face of these choices results not from the technology, but from the fact that we do not yet have the maturity of judgment to know how to make such choices well. In this respect, modern medicine is in an adolescent state of development—aware, like the adolescent, of a wondrous array of newly acquired powers but lacking the judgment born of experience that is necessary for using those powers wisely.

It is possible to shed some light on the precise nature of our distress. The purpose of clinical medicine is to do good for people, and it is in the interest of achieving that good that we allow physicians to do things that would under other circumstances be outlandish and unlawful behavior. Physicians cut people, order them to eat toxic chemicals, manipulate their behavior, and in various other ways perform actions that can be justified only in terms of the larger purpose to which they are directed. We allow this—albeit, often too uncritically—because we want them to achieve the good toward which they aim, and we believe that the distasteful aspects of being a patient are a part of the price that must be paid in order to achieve the benefits. Our concern for doing good—for relieving suffering, prolonging life, enhancing functional abilities, facilitating birth, comforting the bereaved, and all the rest—arises out of our belief that human happiness is of fundamental importance. We want to pursue and enhance it, preferably in the most efficient way.

This outlook is represented in moral philosophy by the ethics of utilitarianism—the view, associated most prominently with the works of John Stuart Mill, that the right thing to do is whatever produces the greatest happiness for the greatest number of people. No moral theory has ever been more powerful or more influential, and we have a widespread tendency to explain and justify our actions in terms of the good that they are intended to produce.

But other values that we hold can conflict with our concern for human happiness. Prominent among them is our respect for the autonomy and dignity of individual persons, and our corresponding concern for the protection of individual rights. The leading proponent of such values among the major philosophers was Immanuel Kant, who had a strict and austere view of morality. Kant held that one must always respect the autonomy of individual persons, and that it is therefore always wrong to view others merely as instruments to be used in the achievement of one's goals. He held, therefore, that one must always treat others as ends unto themselves, and never as means only. Whereas the utilitarian morality directs us to consider the consequences of our actions in deciding what to do, the Kantian morality is unconcerned with consequences. Some kinds of actions, according to the Kantian outlook, are simply wrong, no matter what the benefits might be of performing them. Thus Kant held that it is always wrong, no matter what the circumstances, to break a promise.

This sort of nonconsequentialist morality is quite familiar. The Ten Commandments, for example, are rules of behavior that simply forbid certain kinds of action, such as stealing, without regard to the circumstances under which the act of theft is performed. So the commandment reads, "Thou shalt not steal." It does not read, "Thou shalt not steal, unless you can do more good in the world by stealing than otherwise." Robin Hood was obviously a utilitarian rather than a follower of the Ten Commandments!

The history of moral philosophy is largely concerned with the tension between these two traditions, the consequentialist and nonconsequentialist views of morality. Neither has come to dominate the other, probably because we do care very deeply about the pursuit of good consequences, and yet we believe that there are some limits beyond which that pursuit cannot justifiably take us.

This tension is also prominent in discussion about clinical medicine and medical research. It is respect for the rights of individuals that mainly leads to constraints on the use of human subjects in medical research, and it is concern for the welfare of individuals that mainly motivates the pursuit of medical progress through research. If we were less concerned about protecting the rights of individuals, we could likely make scientific progress at a faster rate, but the progress would not be worth the moral cost. So we limit the use of human subjects in medical research by requiring that the subjects be informed of the nature of the research, and that they consent voluntarily to participate in it. Of course, special problems arise with regard to those who are in no position to consider providing fully informed consent—infants and small children, victims of severe trauma, the seriously retarded or psychotic, and others as well.

The same requirement of informed consent, as a protection of individual rights, applies to clinical practice. Physicians are allowed to behave toward their patients in ways that would not be tolerated as general forms of interpersonal behavior. Such behavior is not justified merely by the fact that the physician intends the patient's good; the physician must have a better justification than that, just as any person must have a better justification than that to intervene in the life or intrude into the body of another person. Nor is it sufficient justification that the physician is a medical practitioner. A license to practice medicine is not a license to go around *imposing* good on people. What justifies the physician's behavior toward a patient, when anything does, is that the physician has a special relationship with that individual patient, according to which it is appropriate to take steps to serve the patient's interests precisely because that is what the patient *wants* done. Under ordinary circumstances—that is, in the absence of emergency, psychosis, or other distorting phenomena—it is the patient's consent that justifies the physician in doing what under other conditions would be abusive, perhaps to the point of felonious assault. What clearer example of this point could there be than the gynecological examination, as we consider how it would be judged if performed outside the context of a doctor-patient relationship? Even if it is a qualified specialist who performs the examination, the absence of consent would transform a standard medical procedure into a criminal action. And it would make no difference that the physician intended the patient's good, or even that the physician was right in thinking that an examination would be good for the patient.

The concept of informed consent, and its application to the interactions in clinical medicine, have given rise to a large and expanding literature, as commentators within and outside medicine try to resolve the various conflicts that swirl around the issue. For there are limits to the extent to which patient consent can be informed, there are often uncertainties about how voluntary it is, and the process of seeking informed consent in clinical contexts has been decried by some commentators as dangerous to health. Yet we have rejected the naive notion that whatever the doctor thinks best is what should be done, and we have entrenched the doctrine of informed consent in the laws regulating medical practice and in the culture of interpersonal expectations within which it is practiced.

The question of who should decide what for whom is difficult in every medical specialty, and that difficulty increases with the advent of increasingly sophisticated technologies. An additional source of tension and potential conflict is present in obstetrical and gynecological practice, however, making ethical conflict even more acute. For it is in such practice that sex-role issues are most sharply etched. Most of the physicians in the specialty are men; all of the patients are women. The stereotypical relationship between male and female shows the male to be the dominant decision maker, especially where technical information is involved, with the female in a comparatively dependent role. Even now, some of the advertisements for automobiles, investment plans, and even wines reflect this pattern. Similarly, the traditional role of the physician is as the wise and beneficent comforter, to whose judgment the patient is subservient. Combine the two phenomena, and a picture emerges of a male physician who soothingly pats his grateful and admiring female patient on the head and says, "Just leave everything to me." The picture is overdrawn, to be sure, yet vestiges of that sort of practice do still remain, and they stand out all the more vividly against the backdrop of increasingly assertive advocacy of the woman's right and responsibility to be informed about and to make autonomous decisions about her own body.

The range of choices that confronts patients is thus growing for two different reasons. First, medical progress is increasing the absolute number of options that are available in the treatment of a patient. Second, patients are coming to play an increasingly active role in selecting among those options. The combined force of these two factors makes it increasingly difficult for physicians to be clear about their own responsibilities and authorities in deciding what should be done. Sometimes, physicians establish an effective relationship with their patients that respects both the expertise of the physician and the autonomy of the patient, avoiding conflict and disappointment. Too often, however, patients and physicians interact to the satisfaction of neither.

Such interaction is exemplified when the physician imposes on the patient a decision that violates the values of that patient; often this occurs because the physician and the patient have different priorities concerning the objectives of treatment. A familiar example is that of the woman in labor who is in pain but wants to remain alert, whose physician decides unilaterally that the relief of her pain is more important than the preservation of her alertness. There may be no medical necessity for such a decision. But the woman and the physician may differ in their attitudes toward pain and toward the importance of mental acuity at the time of childbirth. If treatment is then based on the physician's preferences rather than on what is best for the patient as an autonomous agent, then there has been an imposition of unwanted values on the patient that constitutes an assault on her dignity.

What, then, is to be done? It will not suffice merely to invoke slogans about good medical practice or to sermonize about how good physicians are sensitive to the capacities and aspirations of their patients. Modern medicine is far too complex for that. Instead, it is necessary to acknowledge that ethical considerations must have a central place in medical practice and, therefore, in medical education.

There are two distinct levels of understanding that can be achieved in respect to the ethical problems in clinical medicine, and it is important not to mistake one for the other. The first level is that of being sensitive to the presence of ethical issues, of understanding that conflicts in values have become an ineliminable part of medical practice as technology expands the variety of choices before us, causing us to confront possibilities with respect to which we have no uncontroversial methods of choice. But to recognize the presence of moral dilemmas, even in a sophisticated way, is still to fall short of gaining some competence in dealing with them. It may be better to recognize moral issues than to be blind to them, but it is better still to have some sense of how to deal with them in more than an arbitrary or impulsive way. Achieving that higher level of understanding is a task that lies not only before individual practitioners but before the medical profession as a whole. It is also a task confronting the larger community of patients and the public—the social context within which medicine is practiced.

Of course, there are no simple answers to the moral dilemmas that confront modern medicine. Choices that are simple to make are not the sort we call dilemmas; they are not the sort to cause us to struggle with our consciences, to examine our values, to feel the anxiety that arises out of our ambivalence about what to do. But to acknowledge that the moral challenges of modern medicine are severe is not to despair of confronting them in a reflective and informed way. On the contrary, as I have argued elsewhere, although there is no algorithm for resolving moral disputes or settling moral disagreements, it is nonetheless possible to make some progress toward understanding moral issues in medical practice and how to deal with them.*

---

* Gorovitz, S: *Doctors' dilemmas: Moral conflict and medical care*, Macmillan Publishing Co., New York, 1982.

But that progress will be hard earned, just as progress in medical science is hard earned. Both require patience, tenacity, and an openness to reason, and both are necessary if medical practice is to fulfill its commitment to serving the interests of the patients above all.

As we contemplate a world where obstetrical practice is permeated with electronic marvels, genetic breakthroughs, prenatal surgery, and the like, it is important to remain aware that the entire enterprise arises out of the desire to serve the interests and respect the dignity and aspirations of the people who seek medical care. Where those interests and aspirations are bound up with considerations of birth and family on the one hand and with the prospect of death, disease, and defect on the other, moral issues will unavoidably arise, and their consideration should be an essential part of good medical practice.

SUBMITTED: DECEMBER, 1981
ACCEPTED: DECEMBER, 1981

ANTEPARTUM FETAL HEART RATE TESTS AND INDUCTION OF LABOUR*

Judith Lumley

A screening test should be safe and acceptable for those for whom it is intended. If possible it should be cheap. It should be reliable: that is, there should be acceptable levels of false positive and false negative results. But above all it should have been demonstrated that use of the test has a beneficial effect on the natural history of the disease.[59]

Antepartum fetal monitoring is a screening test with two objectives: to identify the fetus who is already compromised and needs immediate delivery and to identify the fetus who can remain safely in utero. The questions that arise are these: How well does this screening test meet the criteria outlined above? Are all forms of antepartum fetal monitoring equally satisfactory in terms of safety, acceptability, cost, reliability, and contribution to a better outcome? The three forms of monitoring to be reviewed are oxytocin challenge tests, nonstress tests, and unstressed cardiotocography.

Monitoring Fetal Heart Rate and Uterine Activity

Detailed descriptions are readily available.[72] The practical problems associated with the three external fetal heart rate (FHR) monitors include (1) the phonotransducer is subject to interference from ambient sounds; (2) the fetal electrocardiogram is often undetectable in the very small fetus; (3) loss of beat-to-beat (short-term) variability is difficult to detect in the print-out from an ultrasound transducer; and (4) "editing" properties of the system may occasionally cause the fetal heart rate to be recorded at half or double its true value. External monitoring of uterine activity permits recording of the frequency, duration, and relative intensity of the contraction, but it does not measure the actual intra-uterine pressure or the baseline uterine tone.

Women with obesity, hydramnios, or a very small fetus are more difficult to monitor. Most large series report 9% to 10% of unsuccessful or uninterpretable traces (range 1% to 21%).

---

*British spelling is maintained throughout this paper in keeping with the author's country of origin.

Observer Variability in Interpretation of FHR Changes

Aspects of the FHR that may be taken into account in monitoring are the baseline rate, the variability of the baseline rate (both the amplitude and the frequency of changes in the baseline), and the presence of accelerations or decelerations associated with fetal movements or uterine contractions. Five studies of observer variability have been published.

The earliest study classified FHR traces into four categories—normal, suboptimal, decelerative, and terminal—and reported that of 20 recordings, 95% were identically classified by five obstetricians and residents.[100] No other study reported such good agreement.

In 1979, nine experts were asked to rate twelve FHR traces for short-term and long-term variability of the baseline heart rate. Although the authors claim that interobserver agreement was high, no trace was given the same rating by all observers, for either short-term or long-term variability, and one half of the traces were given three different ratings by the nine experts.[19] Another study reported ways of improving reliability for residents, although these were not effective for midwives.[39]

Peck asked five physicians to rate 50 traces from oxytocin challenge tests (OCTs) as positive, negative, or suspicious.[69] Four or more agreed on only 18% of the traces originally read as positive, and only 62% of the traces originally read as negative. Two or more agreed on only 42% of the positive, but 94% of the negative. His conclusion was that "the reading of OCTs even by highly trained obstetricians, although based on objective criteria, is very subjective."[69]

The final study was the most extensive. Five observers scored FHR traces on five criteria. The agreement between them ranged from 63% to 98% and was best for baseline heart rate. There was poor agreement on accelerations. Intraobserver reliability, assessed by rescoring the same traces after a 4-month interval, ranged from 80% to 99%. Overall visual assessments of FHR traces ("eyeballing") as "good," "moderate," or "bad" were much less reliable than scoring, both between and within observers.[96] The authors' conclusions match those of Peck—that the reliability of FHR interpretation leaves a great deal to be desired.

Who is Tested—and When

Common indications for stressed monitoring (oxytocin challenge test/contraction stress test) are hypertension, diabetes, intrauterine growth retardation, previous stillbirth, prolonged pregnancy, maternal cyanotic heart disease, and abnormal estriol or human placental lactogen levels.[29] Unstressed monitoring may be used for the additional indications of antepartum bleeding, multiple pregnancy, polyhydramnios, premature labour, and premature rupture of membranes.[67] Oxytocin for stressed/challenge monitoring may be contraindicated in the latter conditions, as it is in the presence of a uterine scar or an incompetent cervix.

All of the foregoing indications refer to high-risk pregnancies. Recent publications suggest that monitoring is being extended to other groups of women, and two papers recommend universal nonstress testing.[43,89]

Testing begins at the stage in pregnancy when intervention on the grounds of fetal well-being first becomes feasible. Early publications quote 34 weeks' gestation as reasonable, but centres with a neonatal intensive care unit now carry out tests from 28 weeks as a routine.[28]

Oxytocin Challenge Test

The oxytocin challenge test (contraction stress test, OCT/CST)[33,74] looks at the FHR response to the stress of uterine contractions, spontaneous or induced with a controlled infusion of oxytocin. It requires meticulous attention to detail as well as skilled medical or nursing supervision, and it takes 1 to 2 hours to complete. Although early papers differed on such matters as the dose of oxytocin, there is now a standardized protocol for the test and its interpretation.[29] If there is an adequate contraction pattern (that is, at least three uterine contractions in 10 minutes, each lasting for 40 to 60 seconds) in the initial recording periods, however, no oxytocin is necessary.

Three percent to 10% of OCTs are positive; that is, late decelerations of the FHR occur with more than one half of the uterine contractions. A negative test is one in which no late decelerations occur with an adequate contraction pattern. A suspicious or equivocal test is one in which late decelerations occur with less than 50% of the contractions in an adequate contraction pattern. This finding is an indication to repeat the test within 24 to 48 hours. Suspicious tests are at least as common as positive tests.

The other possible test results are failure to obtain an interpretable trace, mentioned earlier as 9% to 10% of tests, and hyperstimulation of the uterus (1% to 3%). The latter (an indication to stop oxytocin) is diagnosed when late decelerations occur with excessive uterine activity: a persistent increase in uterine tone, contractions which last for more than 90 seconds, or contractions closer than every 2 minutes. External monitoring cannot give an accurate estimate of hyperstimulation.

From 1968 to 1980 more than forty series of OCT results were published.* The very earliest tests were "blind," that is, the results were

---

* Full bibliography and summary available from the author.

withheld from the clinicians caring for the patients and not used in patient management. Some workers found positive OCTs to be highly predictive of antepartum stillbirth, severe fetal distress in labour, and neonatal morbidity.[21,78] Elsewhere these results could not be duplicated.[4,14] Despite these inconsistent reports, the OCT became widely used,[36,70,84,85] especially in the United States, without any formal assessment by randomised clinical trial to determine whether the use of the OCT in patient management improved perinatal outcome.

Assessment of OCTs

Some attempts to assess OCTs[63] used inappropriate indicators. It was not surprising, for example, that infants with a positive OCT had a higher caesarean delivery rate than those with a negative OCT when a positive test finding was taken as a reason for immediate intervention.[63] A second measure—the excess perinatal morbidity[36,87] among infants with a positive OCT—could be the result of early intervention as much as severity of underlying chronic fetal distress. Nor could a reduction in the antepartum stillbirth rate[29] be taken at its face value. First, it is vital to ensure that antepartum deaths have not been replaced by neonatal deaths. (A policy of universal caesarean section at the time when births are first registered would completely eliminate antepartum and intrapartum deaths.) Second, in the decade (1970 to 1980) when abdominal delivery nearly tripled in the United States, many high-risk pregnancies would have been terminated prematurely in the absence of OCT results. (One early paper mentioned that all eight patients with positive OCTs had a caesarean on other, clinical grounds.[21])

Comparison of high-risk, OCT-managed pregnancies with the whole obstetrical population fails to take into account the preterm labour category in the general population, who although an ultra-high-risk group, are often poorly identified. High-risk pregnancies managed without OCTs, another comparison group, are characterized by late referral to specialized perinatal centres or lack of antenatal care, making any comparison invalid.

The effectiveness of OCTs in improving the outcome of pregnancy remains unproved.

Two aspects of OCTs have aroused particular comment.

False Positive Tests

A false positive test is one in which a subsequent labour fails to produce fetal distress (late decelerations of the FHR, fetal acidosis, or both). The reported rate of false positive tests is about 40% (range 0% to 100%) among women permitted to labour, who comprise only one third or so of those with positive OCTs, the rest having an elective caesarean section.

Those who do labour after a positive OCT usually have labour induced with oxytocin, a procedure which is known to increase the reporting of late decelerations and fetal distress.[88] Therefore, the very high false positive rate is almost certainly an underestimation. False positives have been attributed to aortocaval compression and reduced uterine blood flow during the test, increased uterine resting pressure during the oxytocin infusion, and the production of contractions that are subtly different from those of true labour.[23]

Whatever the cause, the false positive rate means that the chief risk of OCTs in practice is unnecessary intervention: iatrogenic prematurity and unwarranted caesarean section or induction of labour. The first of these risks was emphasized by Boyd and co-workers, who noted: ''. . . immediate action on one of the three positive results would have needlessly exposed the infant to premature delivery at 33 weeks.''[4] But the true prevalence of unnecessary intervention will not be known until a large randomised clinical trial is carried out, comparing the outcomes for the at-risk fetus managed with and without OCTs. Recent reviews emphasize the need for reevaluation rather than immediate action when the OCT becomes positive.

False Negative Tests

A false negative test is one which is followed by an antepartum stillbirth within 7 days, the conventional interval for retesting. By this criterion, fewer than 1% of tests are falsely negative (3 in 1,000), although about 7% (range 0% to 17%) are falsely negative in terms of fetal distress developing during labour within 7 days of a negative OCT. Extensive reviews of this topic have been published.[58]

Some false negative tests are associated with a sudden deterioration in maternal state (hypotension, diabetic acidosis); some occur in abnormal infants. The two other relatively common causes (abruptio placentae and cord prolapse) are usually discussed as unpredictable accidents, but both might be physiologically possible side effects of oxytocin administration. It is not known whether they occur as often after nonstress testing.

Several centres have reported that the change from negative to positive OCT may be a rapid one, and that the postmature fetus may be particularly liable to sudden deterioration.[68,70]

Some deaths after false negative OCTs highlight the problem of FHR interpretation. Two letters commented that one published negative trace was really equivocal. Another was retrospectively reclassified as suspicious. It is now accepted that one atypical OCT is particularly ominous—one in which there is almost no variability in the baseline FHR and no decelerative response to contractions.[26,35]

The occasional false negative test can only be a problem in situations where OCTs are believed to be an infallible guide and when other signs and symptoms are disregarded in the face of a negative test. The extensive writing on false negatives must arise from the fact that OCTs are now used mainly to reassure the obstetrician that intervention is not yet necessary.[29]

Other hazards of OCTs include hyperstimulation (1% to 3%), which is an additional stress to the at-risk fetus; rupture of uterine scars (theoretical); and accidental induction of labour.[14] The latter has rarely been reported, and a recent review of more than 3,000 tests is reassuring.[6] Bleeding from an undiagnosed placenta praevia has been reported.[60] OCTs have been implicated in the current "epidemic" of neonatal hyperbilirubinaemia.[71] Repeated negative OCTs do not have adverse effects on neonatal behaviour in the first 3 days of life.[86]

Nonstress Tests (NSTs)

Tests of Fetal Reactivity

It was noticed, early in the history of antepartum monitoring, that periodic accelerations of the FHR often occurred in association with fetal movements and that this was a healthy sign, precluding the need for an OCT. A number of workers reanalysed nonstressed FHR portions of the OCT, looking for episodes of such fetal reactivity.[5,46] All reported that, when accelerations were counted as a sign of fetal well-being, the proportion of false positive OCTs was reduced. In the United States, nonstress tests (NSTs) have largely focused on accelerations with fetal movements, in the belief that their presence indicates "intact and responsive central nervous system mechanisms."[67]

NSTs* have not become standardized as OCTs have done. They differ in the duration of the test, the definition of an accelerative (reactive) response, and in the frequency of accelerations needed to qualify as reactive.[57,67] This is one reason why the proportion of nonreactive tests varies so much from one study to another: 35% in one early review of 2,422 tests[20] and 5% in a recent summary of 4,517 tests.[89]

The other reason for the variable proportion of nonreactive tests is that the behavioural state of the fetus affects the occurrence of fetal movements and reactive accelerative responses. It has become customary to include some

---

* Full bibliography and summary available from the author.

form of stimulation after 20 minutes of nonreactive monitoring in an attempt to alter its state.[67] Abdominal manipulation, sound, glucose infusions and eating, or the preliminary phases of an OCT[67] have all been found to shift the fetus into a reactive phase. Maternal factors to be excluded in a nonreactive fetus include unrecognized supine hypotension and many prescribed drugs.[24,40]

False positive NSTs are common (60% with a range of 27% to 77%). The NST has come to be a preliminary screening test for an OCT and, as such, is being extended to low-risk patients as well. One recent paper suggests that preliminary screening should be by ear, with only those fetuses nonreactive on this being referred for NST.[65]

False negative NSTs, like false negative OCTs, are uncommon with 6% (range 2% to 20%) of women having fetal distress in labour within 7 days of a reactive NST. Fetal deaths within 7 days of a reactive NST have been reported as 1 in 1,000 to 7 in 1,000. Failed tests seem to be much less common than with the OCT. Most studies report a failure rate below 2%, although one recorded 13% of unsatisfactory or uninterpretable traces.

Evaluation of NSTs has focused on the question of whether the NST or the OCT is the better predictor of fetal outcome and better sign of present fetal state.[29,67,76] This debate begs the question outlined earlier of whether the use of such screening tests really does improve the outcome of pregnancy. NSTs do not have the specific dangers of oxytocin administration, that is, hyperstimulation, scar rupture, placental separation, and hyperbilirubinaemia.

Unstressed Cardiotocography (CTGs)

In Europe,[24,33,38,43,68,98,100] as in a few North American centres,[42] unstressed tests have taken a different form, with emphasis on several other aspects of the FHR trace (baseline FHR, short-term variability, accelerations or decelerations with contractions, response to fetal movements), than on accelerations (NST) or decelerations (OCT). Although several scoring systems are in use[38,41–43,49,68] they do not differ dramatically.* All end with a three-way classification into normal (reactive, normal baseline, normal variability); abnormal or suspicious (some loss of reactivity, reduced baseline variability, early-mid decelerations); and pathological or severely abnormal or terminal (loss of beat-to-beat variability, late decelerations, absence of reactivity).

Normal women, even ideal women, may have abnormal CTGs (7.2% in one series[97] and 6.8% in another[43]), so it is not surprising that this in-

---

*Complete bibliography and summary available from the author.

termediate category is unhelpful in predicting state at birth. In high-risk patients up to 15% have an abnormal CTG.[38,41]

It might be expected that uninterpretable traces would be more of a problem than with OCTs and NSTs because the FHR trace has to be evaluated with reference to more parameters. Only one study reports the proportion of uninterpretable CTGs: 11%.[49]

Abnormal CTGs have a false positive rate of 14%[42] to 64%,[100] although this is lower when the abnormality is a severe or terminal pattern.[41,101] False negatives by the fetal-distress-in-labour criterion are less common (0.8%[24] to 6%[42]), and by the criterion of death within 7 days of a normal CTG they occur at a rate of 1 in 1,000 cases.

Kubli and co-workers recommend that:

> In non-risk pregnancies, monitoring is done at each antenatal visit starting at 30 weeks gestation. With risk pregnancies monitoring may start earlier in pregnancy, but not before 26/27 weeks and may be repeated weekly, daily or, occasionally, several times a day.[43]

Evaluation of CTGs differs from the evaluation of NSTs and OCTs in only two ways: CTGs have been studied in normal pregnancies,[43,97] and interpretation of CTGs has been assessed comprehensively.[96] Both types of study should reduce the confidence with which CTGs are used as a basis for decision making about intervention in pregnancy.

Overall Assessment of Antenatal FHR Monitoring

How do OCTs, NSTs, and unstressed CTGs compare on the criteria for a successful screening test?

Safety. The main dangers of antenatal FHR monitoring are common to all three methods. They are, apart from as yet unknown long-term effects of repeated exposure to ultrasound, the excess mortality and morbidity of unnecessary intervention. OCTs have, in addition, both contraindications and side effects.

Cost. All three tests need an initial capital outlay and technical maintenance. Monitoring may absorb a great deal of nursing or technician time in antenatal wards and outpatient areas. OCTs are the most expensive in terms of time, and they require high-level supervision.

Acceptability. Antenatal monitoring is highly acceptable to clinicians because it is a reasonably simple test that gives an immediate "answer" on the state of the fetus. In a climate of opinion where it is better to err by commission than by omission, the high false positive rate is acceptable, although the low false negative rate leads to suggestions about more frequent monitoring.

I could find no reports on the acceptability of antenatal monitoring to pregnant women, apart from the occasional mention of "defaulters" from testing. One so far unexplored aspect with major implications for parent acceptability is the high proportion of infants with major abnormalities among those with abnormal FHR traces. A recent paper drew attention to the relationship and pointed out that the abnormal FHR often influenced the decision to perform an emergency caesarean section.[75] A review of the bibliography confirmed that about one in three perinatal deaths was attributed to a major malformation.

Reliability. The problems of observer variation, false negatives, and false positives, which apply to all three tests, have been discussed earlier. None of the tests has a high rating on reliability.

The disagreement about the sequence in which the FHR changes in acute and chronic stress is relevant to whether the NST or the OCT is the better screening test. Flynn and Kelly list the sequence as loss of reactivity, changes in baseline variability, then late decelerations with contractions.[24] Garite and Freeman disagree, reviewing the evidence which supports their belief that loss of reactivity is a late sign, and the presence of late decelerations (especially with oxytocin-induced contractions) "an earlier warning sign of the fetus in jeopardy.[29] However, the absence of late decelerations in the presence of a flat baseline trace is a highly ominous sign.[26,35]

The debates about which test is the best, or which aspect of the FHR to pay most attention to, disregard the physiological evidence that:

> . . . the ultimate response represents the integrated effect of the various local, neural and hormonal factors influencing various cardiovascular functions. Any individual measurement may be influenced by a variety of physiological mechanisms and this must be recognized in interpreting the changes during stress.[83]

It would, in other words, be surprising if a single response, invariably, at all gestations, in all physiological and behavioural states of the fetus, could be recognized as *the* sign of hypoxia.

Beneficial effect on the outcome of the disease. The crucial test of antenatal FHR monitoring is a comparison of women managed with and without monitoring, who are randomly allocated to the two groups and who in all other respects receive identical care.

Four randomised clinical trials of NST in high-risk patients have recently been completed.[31] The four studies, even when combined, were too small to be able to show any effect on perinatal mortality, although in every case the monitored group or the group in which the results of monitoring were available, fared slightly worse: 19 deaths in 796 patients compared with 9 in 784 patients. More than one fourth of these deaths were due to lethal malformations. On all measures of neonatal morbidity (Apgar score, neurological problems [short term], admission to special care, proportion of severely growth-retarded infants), the trial and control groups were remarkably similar.

At present there is no justification for extending the use of NST to all obstetrical patients.

Conclusion

None of the three forms of antepartum FHR monitoring rates very highly as a screening test, on the evidence so far available. The OCT has some additional disadvantages in terms of the contraindications to its use and the relative cost. It is doubtful whether these are outweighed by any greater reliability or more beneficial outcome, on the present evidence.

Antenatal fetal monitoring seems certain to be extended. ("Is any pregnancy low risk?" ask Wilson and Schifrin.)[103] What is uncertain is the direction: multiple biophysical assessments or the tape measure, the stethoscope, and the daily fetal movement chart. The second group have immediate advantages in terms of cost, safety, and acceptability, but *all* screening tests must be assessed on the crucial question: Does the use of this test have a beneficial effect on the outcome of the condition?

Induction of Labour

Induction of labour, the procedure in which labour is initiated artificially before it has begun spontaneously, was first advocated in the early nineteenth century as a way of avoiding obstructed labour. This indication became obsolete, but it was replaced by other situations where continuation of the pregnancy was a clearcut threat to the life or well-being of mother or infant, for example, diabetes and eclampsia. Such medical indications for induction of labour are present in less than 10% of pregnancies.

In the last decade, it has been suggested that a more liberal use of induction would lead to a reduction in perinatal mortality (more specifically, would eliminate hypoxic deaths of mature infants);[52] would increase daytime deliveries, with better supervision of labour and reduced costs of maternity services;[17] and would be more convenient for women and physicians alike.

Rates of Induction of Labour

The controversial nature of indications for induction[79] is demonstrated by the differences between countries (e.g., England and Wales compared with Norway[11]); within one country;[10] between equivalent hospitals in the same city;[48] between public and private patients in the same hospital;[48] or between obstetrical teams in the same hospital.[12] The range is from 5% to 10% at one end up to 50% or more at the other.

Techniques of Induction

Labour may be induced by rupturing the membranes or by administration of oxytocin or prostaglandins. All three techniques are also used for augmentation (also known as enhancement or acceleration) when labour that began spontaneously is stimulated because of unsatisfactory progress. Amniotomy is discussed elsewhere in this volume. Augmentation is beyond the scope of this chapter, but some side effects of induced labours also occur in augmented labours.

Possible Benefits of Induction

Reduced perinatal mortality. Elective induction at, or just before, term would completely eliminate hypoxic deaths of mature infants, it is claimed. Yet antepartum stillbirths in this category account for at most 3 or 4 deaths in 1,000 births,[52,53] so a very large trial would need to be mounted to show a beneficial effect of routine induction on perinatal mortality. Certainly none of the three published trials could be expected to do so, and none did.[15,45,56] A review of birth certificate data for a large sample of New York City births in 1968 detected "a small but significant negative effect" on perinatal mortality of elective induction.[81]

The fact that rising induction rates were associated in time with falling perinatal mortality in several British centres[53,95] is not enough to show a causal relationship, but even this reported relationship has not been found consistently. In one city, induction and active management policies were not associated with any fall in deaths.[12] In another city, a highly satisfactory perinatal mortality was achieved despite an avoidance of elective induction.[64]

The debate illustrates the extreme difficulty of establishing causal relationships from observational data.[93] Two comprehensive reviews discuss causal inference in relation to induced labour,[11,80] and an elegant analysis by Yudkin shows the observational data in one region to be equally compatible with an adverse or a beneficial effect of induction of labour on the fetus.[104]

Planned time of delivery. The distribution of births by day of the week has been altered dramatically by induction policies and active management of labour,[51,82] but there is less agreement on the change in diurnal distribution of births. Some centres report a reduction in night-time work loads,[102] others do not find this to be so.[15] Even when this occurs, the overall work load may not be much less: A 27% fall in births was associated with only an 11% decrease in work load.[102]

Even when more births occur by day and most from Monday to Friday, it is still necessary to provide experienced obstetrical and paediatric supervision all the time. In fact, if the inductees are "normal," out-of-hours work will then have an increasing proportion of abnormal births.[51]

The financial costs and benefits of a high induction rate have been analysed with reference to one of the controlled trials. No significant differences in costs could be detected between the control and induced group.[18]

Convenience. Induction of labour for "convenience," whether this is the mother's or the obstetrician's, is an aspect of the subject where facts are elusive. Induction for the convenience of either party is unlikely to be reported as such, officially. However, Cartwright's study of 2,500 births in Britain found *no* evidence from mothers, midwives, or obstetricians that convenience (alias "social indications") was an important factor there.[10] Evidence for the benefits of a high induction rate is far from convincing.

Possible Hazards of Induction

Iatrogenic prematurity. The main complication of induced labour is the unintended birth of a premature infant.[32,44,55,73] In Sydney, Australia, in 1976 one fourth of all infants admitted to one special care neonatal unit were born after elective induction of labour, and 6 of 23 died.[34] Flaksman and others reported from Ohio that inappropriate induction severely affected 1.6 infants for every 1,000 live births, with subsequent mortality, morbidity, and emotional and financial costs.[23] Lesser degrees of prematurity may be even more common.[2,47]

The prevalence of iatrogenic prematurity will be affected by the quality of obstetrical care as well as the induction rate. One centre excluded all patients in whom the clinical estimation of gestation might have been inaccurate—and was left with 16% of the obstetrical population.[56] In addition to careful clinical assessment, the routine use of tests for fetal maturity (ultrasonic examination, amniocentesis, and estimation of lecithin/ sphingomyelin ratio) before induction has been advocated,[23,34] although these, of course, have their own risks to be taken into account as well.

Increased use of other interventions. The secular trend in induced labours has occurred at the same time as an increase in forceps deliveries, epidural anaesthetics, and caesarean sections,[22] but as with perinatal mortality, the association may not be causal. The three randomised trials[15,45,56] found no effect of induction on other interventions, and one retrospective study of mature infants admitted to special care nurseries failed to implicate induction in the sequence of events leading to admission.[1] However, a case-control study of 200 matched pairs of women did confirm an association of elective induction with an increase in fetal heart rate monitoring, epidural anaesthesia, forceps delivery, caesarean section, and the birth of infants needing special resuscitation.[105]

Failed induction of labour, resulting in caesarean section, is an example of a direct effect of induction on other interventions. It is rarely identified as such, but usually recorded as one of the forms of "failure to progress" in labour.

Fetal distress. Oxytocin administration can stress the fetus by causing hypertonic contractions of the uterus, as mentioned earlier, but even with normal contractions it is associated with more frequent late decelerations of the fetal heart rate. In Oxford in the early 1970s, a rising induction rate, from 32% to 55% of labours, was related to an increase in emergency caesarean sections for fetal distress.[3]

Prostaglandins can also cause fetal distress and hypercontractility.[30,94] Fetal death has been reported after the use of prostaglandins overnight to ripen the cervix for induction.[77]

Neonatal jaundice. Disagreement about the role of oxytocin and induction in the recent pandemic of neonatal jaundice continues.[80] It is likely to be multifactorial,[37] with some factors (e.g., oxytocin, head pressure after membrane rupture, and mild prematurity) being synergistic. Two of the randomised trials detected an effect of induction, which is stronger evidence of a causal relationship than the observation of an association.[15,56] Jaundice has been recorded after prostaglandin inductions,[8] although not in all studies.[13] When induction leads to epidural anaesthesia or forceps delivery, these procedures may also contribute to jaundice.[80]

Hazards to the mother. 1. Pain is greater when labour is induced. A National Childbirth Trust survey in Britain found that two thirds of the women whose first labour had been spontaneous and second labour induced found the second, induced labour to be more painful. When both labours were spon-taneous, only 4% found the second labour more painful than the first. More women in this study (92% compared with 50%) were given drugs for relief of pain in induced than spontaneous labour.[91] Cartwright's large sample con-firmed the greater use of drugs.[10]

When control of pain by prepared childbirth techniques is important to the woman, induction and the subsequent rapid, painful labour can be a disturbing blow to her self-confidence and self-esteem. The effects of drugs on maternal and infant behaviour are beyond the scope of this chapter.

2. Postpartum haemorrhage is commoner after induced labour, even when corrected for method of delivery and parity.[7] Oxytocin is implicated in this effect, and there is as yet no information on haemorrhage after pro-staglandin induction.

3. The antidiuretic effect of oxytocin can lead to hyponatraemia (with convulsions) in mother and infant, especially when oxytocin is administered in large volumes of electrolyte-poor fluid.[54,90]

4. One German paper reported an increase in third degree tears.[92]

5. Oakley's study of the sociology of childbirth in normal primigravidas raises the disturbing possibility that induction, as part of a "controlled" birth, contributes to postpartum depression.[62]

Separation of infant and mother. The neonatal complications of induc-tion, that is, prematurity, operative delivery, fetal distress, and jaundice, will all lead to separation from the mother for special care.[80] Some women are separated "pharmacologically" rather than physically, their conscious state being adversely affected by the drugs they have been given for pain relief. The National Childbirth Trust found that 42% of mothers were separated from their infants after induced labours.[91] Lack of contact after birth may possibly interfere with the establishment of mother-infant bonding.[9]

Acceptability of Induction

It has been suggested by editorial writers of medical journals that induc-tion of labour is highly acceptable to all except a tiny minority of women espousing a "natural" rather than a "medical" paradigm of birth. However 2,000 women in Britain, randomly sampled from those who gave birth in mid-1975, did not find induction acceptable: 78% of those who had an in-duced labour and 95% of those who had a spontaneous labour would not want an induced labour in the future.[10]

Follow-up of Children Born After Elective Induction

Three neonatal studies differ in the form of assessment, the groups compared, and the findings. One randomised clinical trial of induction found no differences in neonates on the first or fifth day, assessed by the Brazelton scale.[45] Another study compared neurophysiological responses after spontaneous, oxytocin-induced, and prostaglandin-induced labours. The latter differed significantly from the spontaneous onset group in terms of "resting brain activity."[16] The third study found subtle differences in infant behaviour that were still present a few months after birth. These were associated with oxytocin use but not with the prostaglandins.[66]

Psychomotor development was assessed in two studies of preschool children. One showed no ill effects of prostaglandin induction at 30 months of age.[94] The other reviewed children at 23 to 62 months and found 11 of 156 with developmental problems. Two of them might possibly have been related to oxytocin induction, none to prostaglandins.[27]

Two more long-term studies have failed to find adverse effects on intelligence or perceptual-motor performance at 4 and 5 years of age.[50,61] Neither included any preterm infants, so the question is still unresolved as to whether prematurity plus induction adversely affects behaviour or learning, particularly in the context of inadequate parental caretaking.

Conclusion

The possible dangers of any procedure must be taken into account, especially when its use is advocated for large numbers of healthy women and their babies. Induction of labour, although potentially a reliable and life-saving procedure, is not free from risk. Indeed, from the circumstantial evidence available, reviewed elsewhere[11,80] and summarized earlier, it seems that as generally practiced, the costs of induction may well outweigh the benefits. *The Lancet*'s editorial is fair comment:

> The timing of spontaneous delivery is controlled by complex mechanisms which are still incompletely understood, despite intensive research, and which have as their end point the delivery of the young at a stage of maturity at which survival of the newborn is most likely. Is it correct to advocate wholesale interference with this delicately balanced physiological process?[17]

However, the following question has greater implications for research workers, obstetricians, and consumers:

How did it happen that a procedure which had not been carefully evaluated, which involved considerable costs and hazards, and was disliked by child-bearing women, came to be used so widely and accepted uncritically?[10]

REFERENCES

1. Adelstein P, Fedrick J, Howat P, et al. Obstetric practice and infant morbidity. *Br J Obstet Gynaecol* 84:721–725, 1977.

2. Blacow M, Smith M N, Graham M, et al. Induction of labour. *Lancet* 1:217, 1975.

3. Bonnar J. Selective induction of labour. *Br Med J* 1:651–652, 1976.

4. Boyd I E, Chamberlain G V, Fergusson I L. The oxytocin stress test and the isoxsuprine placental transfer test in the management of suspected placental insufficiency. *J Obstet Gynaecol Br Commonw* 81:120–125, 1974.

5. Braly P, Freeman R K. The significance of fetal heart rate reactivity with a positive oxytocin challenge test. *Obstet Gynecol* 50:689–693, 1977.

6. Braly P, Freeman R K. Premature labour and the oxytocin challenge test (quoted in Garite and Freeman, *qv*, 29).

7. Brinsden P R, Clark A D. Postpartum haemorrhage after induced and spontaneous labour. *Br Med J* 2:855–856, 1978.

8. Calder A A, Moar V A, Ounsted M K, et al. Increased bilirubin levels in neonates after induction of labor by intravenous prostaglandin E^2 or oxytocin. *Lancet* 2:1339–1342, 1974.

9. Campbell S B G, Taylor P M. Bonding and attachment: Theoretical issues. *Semin Perinatol* 3:3–13, 1979.

10. Cartwright A. *The dignity of labour? A study of childbearing and induction.* London, Tavistock Press, 1979.

11. Chalmers I, Richards M P M. Intervention and causal inference in obstetric practice. In Chard, T Richards M P M (eds). *Benefits and hazards of the new obstetrics.* London, Spastics International Medical Publications, 1977.

12. Chalmers I, Zlosnik J E, Johns K A, et al. Obstetric practice and outcome of pregnancy in Cardiff residents 1965–1973. *Br Med J* 1:735–738, 1976.

13. Chew W C. Neonatal hyperbilirubinaemia: A comparison between prostaglandin E$_2$ and oxytocin inductions. *Br Med J* 2:679–680, 1977.

14. Christie G B, Cudmore D W. The oxytocin challenge test. *Am J Obstet Gynecol* 118:327–330, 1974.

15. Cole R A, Howie P W, Macnaughton M C. Elective induction of labor: A randomized prospective trial. *Lancet* 1:767–770, 1975.

16. Crowell D H, Sharma S D, Philip A G S, et al. Effects of induction of labour on the neurophysiologic functioning of newborn infants. *Am J Obstet Gynecol* 136:48-53, 1980.

17. Editorial. A time to be born. *Lancet* 2:1183, 1974.

18. Engleman S R, Hilland M A, Howie, P W, et al. An analysis of the economic implications of induction of labour at term. *Commun Med* 1:191–198, 1979.

19. Escarcena L, McKinney R D, Depp R. Fetal baseline heart rate variability estimation. *Am J Obstet Gynecol* 136:615–621, 1979.

20. Evertson L R, Paul R H. Antepartum fetal heart rate testing: the non-stress test. *Am J Obstet Gynecol* 132:895–900, 1978.

21. Ewing D E, Farina J R, Otterson W N. Clinical application of the oxytocin challenge test. *Obstet Gynecol* 43:563-566, 1974.
22. Fedrick J, Yudkin P. Obstetric practice in the Oxford Record Linkage area study 1965-72. *Br Med J* 1:738-740, 1976.
23. Flaksman R J, Vollman J H, Benfield D G. Iatrogenic prematurity due to elective termination of the uncomplicated pregnancy: A major perinatal health care problem. *Am J Obstet Gynecol* 132:885-888, 1978.
24. Flynn A M, Kelly J. Evaluation of fetal wellbeing by antepartum fetal heart monitoring. *Br Med J* 1:936-939, 1977.
25. Flynn A M, Kelly J, O'Conor M. Unstressed antepartum CTG in the management of the fetus suspected of growth retardation. *Br J Obstet Gynaecol* 86:106-110, 1979.
26. Freeman R K, James J. Clinical experience with the oxytocin challenge test. II: An ominous atypical pattern. *Obstet Gynecol* 46:255-259, 1975.
27. Friedman E A, Sachtleben M R, Wallace A K. Infant outcome following labor induction. *Am J Obstet Gynecol* 133:718-722, 1979.
28. Gabbe S G, Freeman R D, Geobelsmann U. Evaluation of the contraction stress test before 33 weeks gestation. *Obstet Gynecol* 52:649-652, 1978.
29. Garite T J, Freeman R K. Antepartum stress test monitoring. *Clin Obstet Gynecol* 6:295-307, 1979.
30. Gonzalez-Merlo J, Ribas-Barba J, Guerra T, et al. Fetal effects of prostaglandin induction of labour. In Karim S M M (ed). *Obstetric and gynaecological uses of prostaglandins.* Asian Federation of Obstetrics and Gynaecology, First Inter-Congress, 1976. Lancaster; M. T. P. Press, 1976.
31. Grant A, Mohide P. Screening tests and diagnostic procedures in antenatal care. In Enkin M, Chalmers I (eds). *Effectiveness and satisfaction in antenatal care.* London, Spastics International Medical Publications, 1982.
32. Hack M, Fanaroff A A, Klaus M H, et al. Neonatal respiratory distress following elective delivery: A preventable disease? *Am J Obstet Gynecol* 126:43-47, 1976.
33. Hammacher K, Hueter K A, Bokelmann J, et al. Foetal heart frequency and perinatal condition of the foetus and newborn. *Gynaecologia* 166:349-360, 1968.
34. Henderson-Smart D J, Storey B. Perinatal implications of the respiratory distress syndrome. *Med J Aust* 2:857-859, 1976.
35. Homburg R, Insler V. Loss of beat-to-beat variability and a negative oxytocin challenge test: An ominous prognostic sign. *Int J Gynaecol Obstet* 17:159-163, 1979.
36. Huddleston J F, Sutcliff G, Carney F E, et al. Oxytocin challenge test for antepartum assessment. *Am J Obstet Gynecol* 135:609-614, 1979.
37. Jeffares M J. A multifactorial survey of neonatal jaundice. *Br J Obstet Gynaecol* 84:452-455, 1977.
38. Jordan B, Hoheisel M. Erste Erfahrungen mit dem Beurteilungsschema nach Fischer für das antepartale Kardiotokogramm. *Geburtsh Frauenheilk* 37:781-787, 1977.
39. Kariniemi V. Evaluation of fetal heart rate variability by a visual semiquantitative method and by a quantitative statistical method with the use of a mini-computer. *Am J Obstet Gynecol* 130:588-590, 1978.
40. Keegan K A, Paul R H, Broussard P M, et al. Antepartum fetal heart rate testing. III: The effect of phenobarbital on the nonstress test. *Am J Obstet Gynecol* 133:579-580, 1979.
41. Keirse M J N C, Trimbos J B. Assessment of antepartum cardiotocograms in high risk pregnancy. *Br J Obstet Gynaecol* 87:261-269, 1980.
42. Krebs H B, Petres R E. Clinical application of a scoring system for evaluation of antepartum fetal heart rate monitoring. *Am J Obstet Gynecol* 130:765-772, 1978.
43. Kubli F, Boos R, Rüttgers H, et al. Antepartum fetal heart rate monitoring. In Beard R W, Campbell S (eds). *The current status of fetal heart rate monitoring and ultrasound in obstetrics.* London, Royal College of Obstetricians and Gynaecologists. 1977.

44. Le Guennec J C, Bard H, Teasdale F, et al. Elective delivery and the neonatal respiratory distress syndrome. *Can Med Assoc J* 122:307–309, 1980.

45. Leijon I, Finnström O, Hedenskog S, et al. Spontaneous labour and elective induction—a prospective randomized study: Behavioral assessment and neurological examination in the newborn period. *Acta Paediatr Scand* 68:553–560, 1979.

46. Lin C -C, Moawad A H, River P, et al. An OCT reactivity classification to predict fetal outcome. *Obstet Gynecol* 56:17–23, 1980.

47. Liston W A, Campbell A J. Dangers of oxytocin induced labour to fetuses. *Br Med J* 3:606–607, 1974.

48. Lumley J. Patterns of obstetric intervention: Tasmania and Victoria. *New Doctor* 15:27–29, 1980.

49. Lyons E R, Bylsma-Howell M, Shamsi S, et al. A scoring system for nonstresed antepartum fetal heart rate monitoring. *Am J Obstet Gynecol* 133:242–246, 1979.

50. McBride W G, Lyle J G, Black B, et al. A study of five year old children born after elective induction of labour. *Med J Aust* 2:456–459, 1977.

51. Macfarlane A. Variations in number of births and perinatal mortality by day of week in England and Wales. *Br Med J* 2:1670–1673, 1978.

52. McIlwaine G M, MacNaughton M C, Richards I D G, et al. A study of perinatal deaths in Glasgow. *Health Bull* 32:103–107, 1974.

53. McNay M B, McIlwaine G M, Howie P W, et al. Perinatal deaths: Analysis by clinical cause to assess value of induction of labour. *Br Med J* 1:347–350, 1977.

54. McKenna P, Shaw R W. Hyponatremic fits in oxytocin-augmented labours. *Int J Gynaecol Obstet* 17:250–252, 1979.

55. Maisels M J, Rees R, Marks K, et al. Elective delivery of the term fetus: An obstetrical hazard. *J A M A* 238:2036–2039, 1977.

56. Martin D H, Thompson W, Pinkerton J H M, et al. A randomized controlled trial of selective planned delivery. *Br J Obstet Gynaecol* 85:109–113, 1978.

57. Mendenhall H W, O'Leary J A, Phillips K O. The nonstress test: The value of a single acceleration in evaluating the fetus at risk. *Am J Obstet Gynecol* 136:87–91, 1980.

58. Neuhoff, SD, Gal D, Tancer M L. False negative oxytocin challenge test result: Review. *N Y State J Med* 79:1537–1540, 1979.

59. Newcombe R, Fedrick J, Chalmers I. Antenatal identification of patients "at risk" of preterm labour. In Anderson A, Beard R, Brudenell J M, et al. (eds). *Pre-term labour. Proceedings 5th Study Group of the R C O G, 1977.* London, Royal College of Obstetricians and Gynaecologists, 1978.

60. Ng K H, Wong W P. Risk of haemorrhage in oxytocin stress test. *Br Med J* 2:698–699, 1976.

61. Niswander K R, Turoff B B, Romans J. Developmental status of children delivered through elective induction of labour. *Obstet Gynecol* 27:15, 1966.

62. Oakley A. *Women confined.* New York, Schocken Books, Inc., 1980.

63. Odendaal H J. The fetal and labour outcome of 102 positive oxytocin contraction stress tests. *Obstet Gynecol* 54:591–596, 1979.

64. O'Driscoll K, Caroll C J, Coughlan M. Selective induction of labour. *Br Med J* 4:727–729, 1975.

65. O'Leary J A, Mendenhall H W, Andrinopoulos G G. Comparison of auditory versus electronic assessment of antenatal fetal welfare. *Obstet Gynecol* 56:244–246, 1980.

66. Ounsted M K, Boyd P A, Hendrick A M, et al. Induction of labour by different methods in primiparous women. II: Neurobehavioral status of the infants. *Early Hum Develop* 2(3):241–253, 1978.

67. Paul R H, Keegan K A. Nonstress antepartum fetal monitoring. *Clin Obstet Gynecol* 6:351–358, 1979.

68. Pearson J F, Weaver J B. A six point scoring system for antenatal cardiotocographs. *Br J Obstet Gynaecol* 85:321–327, 1978.

69. Peck T M. Physicians' subjectivity in evaluating oxytocin challenge tests. *Obstet Gynecol* 56:13–16, 1980.

70. Peck T M. Electronic monitoring evidence of fetal distress in high risk pregnancies. *J Reprod Med* 24:103–108, 1980.

71. Peleg D, Goldman J A. Oxytocin challenge test and neonatal hyperbilirubinaemia. *Lancet* 2:1026, 1976.

72. Pillay S K, Chik L, Sokol R J, et al. Fetal monitoring: A guide to understanding the equipment. *Clin Obstet Gynecol* 22:571–582, 1979.

73. Pinkerton J H M, Martin D H, Thompson W. Selective planned induction in conditions of civil strife. *Lancet* 1:197–198, 1975.

74. Posé S V, Castillo J B, Mora-Rojas E O, et al. Test of fetal tolerance to induced contractions for the diagnosis of chronic fetal distress. *Int J Gynaecol Obstet* 8:142–143, 1970.

75. Powell-Phillips W D, Towell M E. Abnormal fetal heart rate associated with congenital abnormalities. *Br J Obstet Gynaecol* 87:270–274, 1980.

76. Pratt D, Diamond F, Yen H, et al. Fetal stress and nonstress tests: An analysis and comparison of their ability to identify fetal outcome. *Obstet Gynecol* 54:419–423, 1979.

77. Quinn MA, Murphy AJ. Fetal death following extra-amniotic prostaglandin gel. Report of two cases. *Br J Obstet Gynaecol* 88:650–651, 1981.

78. Ray M, Freeman R, Pine S, et al. Clinical experience with the oxytocin challenge test. *Am J Obstet Gynecol* 114:1–9, 1972.

79. Richards M P M. Innovation in medical practice: Obstetricians and the induction of labour in Britain. *Soc Sci Med* 9:595–602, 1975.

80. Richards M P M. The induction and acceleration of labour: Some benefits and complications. *Early Hum Develop* 1:3–17, 1977.

81. Rindfuss R R, Gortmaker S L, Ladinsky J L. Elective induction and stimulation of labour and the health of the infant: Evidence from New York City. *Am J Public Health* 68:872–877, 1978.

82. Rindfuss R R, Ladinsky J L, Coppock E, et al. Convenience and the occurrence of births: Induction of labour in the United States and Canada. *Int J Health Serv* 9:439–460, 1979.

83. Rudolph A M, Itskovitz J, Iwamoto H, et al. Fetal cardiovascular responses to stress. *Semin Perinatol* 5:109–121, 1981.

84. Sanchez-Ramos J E, Sandoval C, Llusia J B. The oxytocin challenge test in the prognosis of high risk labor. *Z Geburtsh Perinatol* 180:220–224, 1976.

85. Sandenbergh H A, Odendaal H J. Clinical experience with the contraction stress test. *S Afr Med J* 51:660-663, 1977.

86. Scanlon J W, Suzuki K, Shea E, et al. Clinical and neurobehavioral effects of repeated intrauterine exposure to oxytocin: A prospective study. *Am J Obstet Gynecol* 132:294–296, 1978.

87. Scanlon J W, Suzuki K, Shea E, et al. A prospective study of the oxytocin challenge test and newborn neurobehavioral outcome. *Obstet Gynecol* 54:6–11, 1979.

88. Schifrin B S. Fetal heart rate patterns following epidural anaesthesia and oxytocin infusion during labour. *J Obstet Gynaecol Br Commonw.* 79:332-339, 1972.

89. Schifrin B S, Foye G, Amato J, et al. Routine fetal heart rate monitoring in the antepartum period. *Obstet Gynecol* 54:21–25, 1979.

90. Schwartz R H, Jones R W A. Transplacental hyponatraemia due to oxytocin. *Br Med J* 1:152–153, 1978.

91. *Some mothers' experiences of induced labour.* In Kitzinger, S. (ed). London. National Childbirth Trust, 1975.

92. Stockhammer P, Villinger C, Haensel W, et al. Kritische Beobachtungen über den Dammris. III. *Geburtshilfe Frauenheilk* 36:759–763, 1976.

93. Susser M W. *Causal thinking in the health sciences.* London, Oxford University Press, 1973.

94. Thiery M, Amy J. Perinatal effects of prostaglandins used for induction of labour. In Karim S S S (ed). *Obstetric and gynaecological uses of prostaglandins.* Asian Federation of Obstetrics and Gynaecology, First Inter-congress, 1976. Lancaster, M.T.P. Press, 1976.

95. Tipton R H, Lewis B V. Induction of labour and perinatal mortality. *Br Med J* 1:391, 1975.

96. Trimbos J B, Keirse M J N C. Observer variability in assessment of antepartum cardiotocograms. *Br J Obstet Gynaecol* 85:900–906, 1978.

97. Trimbos J B, Keirse M J N C. Significance of antepartum cardiotocography in normal pregnancy. *Br J Obstet Gynaecol* 85:907–913, 1978.

98. Tushuizen P B T, Stoot J E G M, Ubachs J M H. Abnormal antepartum cardiotocograms in patients with placental insufficiency. *Am J Obstet Gynecol* 119:638–647, 1974.

99. Tushuizen P B T, Stoot J E G M, Ubachs J M H. Clinical experience in nonstressed antepartum cardiotocography. *Am J Obstet Gynecol* 128:507–513, 1977.

100. Visser G H, Huisjes H J. Diagnostic value of the unstressed antepartum cardiotocogram. *Br J Obstet Gynaecol* 84:321–326, 1977.

101. Visser G H, Redman C W G, Huisjes H J, et al. Nonstressed antepartum heart rate monitoring: Implications of decelerations after spontaneous contractions. *Am J Obstet Gynecol* 138:429–435, 1980.

102. Williams S M. Effect of planned deliveries on labour ward staffing. *Midwife Health Visit Commun Nurse* 12:387–389, 1976.

103. Wilson R W, Schifrin B S. Is any pregnancy low risk? *Obstet Gynecol* 55:653–656, 1980.

104. Yudkin P. Problems in assessing effects of induction of labour on perinatal mortality. *Br J Obstet Gynaecol* 83:603–607, 1976.

105. Yudkin P, Frumar A M, Anderson A B, et al. A retrospective study of induction of labour. *Br J Obstet Gynaecol* 86:257–265, 1979.

SUBMITTED: APRIL, 1981
REVISED & ACCEPTED: JULY, 1982

AMNIOCENTESIS

Irwin H. Kaiser

Amniocentesis in human beings at the present time is a procedure that is conducted for diagnosis and for treatment. Early in the development of the technique, it was found possible to do it throughout pregnancy, but its use in the first trimester has been abandoned because of an unacceptable incidence of complications. In the second trimester the therapeutic use of amniocentesis is at present entirely theoretical. Its major employment is for genetic diagnosis and for purposes of abortion. In the third trimester, amniocentesis is carried out to assist in decisions concerning fetal welfare.

Genetic Diagnosis

Genetic diagnosis by amniocentesis may be accomplished by growing the cells shed into the amniotic fluid from the surface of the fetus in tissue culture. These cells can then be studied in two ways. One procedure is an analysis of their chromosome complement that makes it possible to diagnose conditions associated with abnormalities of chromosomes, such as Down's syndrome, Klinefelter's syndrome, Potter's syndrome, and several other relatively uncommon abnormalities. These are associated with either structural defects of individual chromosomes or the presence of excessive numbers of chromosomes. With rare exceptions polysomy of chromosomes occurs increasingly as maternal age increases, and it is for this reason that the greatest use of amniocentesis has been among women in the last decade of reproductive life, that is, past the age of 35 years.

The other procedure is the study of the cells grown from amniotic fluid to determine the presence or absence of specific enzyme systems that are associated with congenital metabolic abnormalities. When either of these studies is done, it is important to study the cells which have presumably been grown from the amniotic fluid of the fetus to be certain that they have not been obtained from the mother by error. Efficient identification techniques are presently available to make this distinction.

In addition, the fluid itself can be studied for the presence or absence of particular chemicals associated with metabolic disorders and with certain anatomical defects. An example of the latter is the presence of excessive quantities of alpha-fetoprotein when the closure of the fetus's central nervous system fails to complete itself. The nervous system of the embryo begins as an open tube, which later closes over. The failure of this closure allows excessive amounts of alpha-fetoprotein to enter the amniotic fluid and from the amniotic fluid to enter the mother's bloodstream. Determination of excessive alpha-fetoprotein in maternal serum has been used as a screening procedure in high-risk populations such as those in Northern England and Scotland. Those pregnant women with abnormally high serum alphafetoprotein are then studied further. The combination of amniocentesis for the determination of amniotic fluid alpha-fetoprotein and diagnostic ultrasound makes possible the accurate diagnosis of almost all major neural tube defects.

The accuracy of diagnosis of genetic disorders such as these has been approximated by most authors as 99%. Since some cytological and biochemical procedures are in the advancing edge of new technology, however, errors have been and continue to be made, both in failure to diagnose abnormalities that are present and in the incorrect affirmative diagnosis of abnormalities that are absent. In the best laboratories there is awareness of these pitfalls, and much effort is being devoted to reducing the incidence of erroneous diagnoses.

Pregnancy Termination

Amniocentesis for abortion principally involves the administration of substances into the amniotic fluid that have the effect of killing the fetus, the effect of stimulating sufficient uterine activity to result in abortion, or both. A considerable variety of such substances has been used, all of which involve some risk to the mother. For this reason, at the present time, common practice is to combine induction of fetal death and labor by amniocentesis with other modalities, such as the use of laminaria to dilate the cervix and of intravenous oxytocin to stimulate uterine activity.

In two remarkable cases that have been formally reported in the medical literature, amniocentesis has been employed to kill the abnormal member of a twin pair. In one instance a diagnosis of Hurler's syndrome had been made on a twin, and in the other instance a diagnosis of Down's syndrome.[16] In both cases cardiac puncture of the abnormal twin was accomplished, and the twin's death was brought about by withdrawal of blood from the heart. In both instances the normal twin survived. Abortion by this technique is not without risk to the normal twin, since in some instances of monozygotic twinning the two fetuses have a common circulation at the placenta.[7] The fact that the twins are discordant does not provide complete assurance that they are dizygotic.[24]

At the present time, there exists only the theoretical possibility of undertaking treatment of genetic abnormalities by amniocentesis in the second trimester.

Pulmonary Maturity

In the third trimester the usefulness of amniocentesis has been in other directions. The commonest diagnostic use is the withdrawal of fluid to study it for the presence of the several chemicals that are involved in the maturity of the lungs. Before these biochemical techniques were developed, a number of other substances in amniotic fluid were studied because they correlated with maturity in general, for example, studies for fat derived from vernix caseosa, which is ordinarily present only in the last several weeks of pregnancy, and for the concentration of creatinine in the fluid. However, since the measurement of these substances does not give the desired level of predictability in regard to lung function, which is probably the critical event in the survival of the fetus after birth, in recent years the greatest attention has been directed toward the determination of the ratio between lecithin and sphingomyelin and, more recently, the amount of phosphatidyl glycerol in amniotic fluid. As term approaches, more and more lecithin is produced, and its concentration is generally expressed as the L/S ratio. The efficiency of lecithin in bringing about normal pulmonary function after birth is affected by the presence of phosphatidyl glycerol. It is clear, however, that phosphatidyl glycerol in the absence of lecithin is not effective, nor is lecithin in the absence of phosphatidyl glycerol. It is possible to have a high L/S ratio and, nevertheless, an infant who suffers from respiratory distress syndrome. Studies of both these materials allows a very high level of predictability of restricted pulmonary function in the newborns.

The problem of predicting pulmonary maturity arises most frequently in the context of decisions to perform elective cesarean sections. Since the commonest indication for this surgery in the United States is the history of a previous cesarean section, it has been recommended that every such patient have an amniocentesis and a study of the L/S ratio. Some authors, aware that this procedure is not without risk, have urged that the decision as to the timing of repeat cesarean section might better be made by early prenatal care, careful recording of the onset of fetal movements, ultrasound examination halfway through pregnancy when measurement of the biparietal diameter correlates best with gestational age, and the use of amniocentesis only in doubtful situations.[10] It is also clear, however, that the woman who has previously undergone a cervical cesarean section can be allowed to go into labor even if a repeat cesarean section is planned.[3] The lowest incidence of avoidable respiratory distress syndrome due to prematurity would be achieved by having all such patients experience labor before the cesarean section is performed. Amniocentesis for the diagnosis of pulmonary maturity could be limited to the occasional case where there is a complication of pregnancy probably necessitating premature delivery, and some doubt exists as to the ability of the fetus to survive if premature delivery is carried out. It is not yet clear whether some of these complications may not actually enhance the neonate's lung maturity and make the amniocentesis unnecessary.

It has been suggested that among patients who have premature rupture of the membranes, which may be associated with intrauterine infection, amniocentesis could be used for bacterial culture and study of the fluid for the presence of inflammatory cells to allow an earlier diagnosis of chorioamnionitis. Careful study of this problem has demonstrated that there is probably no clinical advantage to this technique when it is compared with other modalities for the diagnosis of chorioamnionitis.[11]

Blood Group Isoimmunization

Amniocentesis is extremely useful in the management of patients with blood group isoimmunization. In this situation the mother forms antibodies against the red blood cells of her fetus. This can be diagnosed by examining maternal blood. The antibodies cross the placenta into the fetus and act to destroy the fetus's red cells. The fetus becomes anemic and excretes hemoglobin breakdown products into the amniotic fluid. By studying the concentration of these products, the principal one being bilirubin, an estimate can be made of the severity of fetal anemia. This procedure is carried out in some severe cases as early as the end of the second trimester, but surely is indicated by the 28th to 30th week of pregnancy and as often as needed thereafter. In some fetuses, analysis of amniotic fluid shows so much damage that the fetus would not survive long enough for its lungs to be sufficiently mature for life outside the uterus. This fetus can then be treated by intrauterine blood transfusion, which is done by amniocentesis techniques, injecting blood directly into the fetus. This has been performed successfully many hundreds of times. If the severity of the process is not too great, the pregnancy can simply be observed until lung maturity is present; the fetus is then delivered and transfusion carried out directly after birth. In even milder cases it is necessary only to do amniocentesis to corroborate the fact that the process is not sufficiently severe to result in stillbirth.

Intrauterine Procedures

Intrauterine transfusion is a subset of amniocentesis, and at present has become materially simpler to carry out with the use of real-time ultrasonography. Fortunately, the use of hyperimmune human anti-D globulin, commercially known as RhoGAM, has greatly reduced the incidence of sensitized women, and therefore of affected infants, so that as the technology has advanced the need to employ it has decreased significantly.

Clearly there ought to be broad possibilities for intrauterine treatment of other conditions. Self-evident is the administration of antibiotics in the event of intrauterine infection. However, from a practical standpoint this has not been sufficiently effective to replace prompt delivery and direct treatment of the infant in an uninfected environment. For a number of years, there has been interest in the use of corticoids to accelerate lung maturity in fetuses expected to be born prematurely. By and large, the steroids have been administered to the mother, but in some studies the steroids have been administered directly into amniotic fluid and, hence directly to the infant. This route of administration does not seem to be in any way superior to the administration of the same drugs to the mother. A few experimental studies have also been conducted on the use of such drugs as atropine administered to the fetus in utero in the treatment of bradycardia, but once again it has been difficult to demonstrate any really desirable clinical effect.

Amniocentesis has been used successfully in the treatment of patients whose fetuses produce vastly excessive amounts of amniotic fluid. This is occasionally extreme even in the presence of a normal fetus. Pitkin has reported an instance of such polyhydramnios in which almost 12 liters of amniotic fluid was removed by 27 amnionteses over a period of 57 days, with survival of the newborn.[25] Many other less dramatic cases have been treated by smaller numbers of amnionteses for the withdrawal of the excessive fluid.

Several instances of successful efforts to treat other fetal abnormalities such as urinary obstruction, hydrocephalus, and excess pleural fluid have recently been reported.[2,18,27,28] It is too soon to say how frequently there will be occasion for such procedures or how effective this intervention will be.

Complications

The usefulness of any diagnostic and therapeutic modality must be measured against its risks. In the late 1940s and all through the 1950s, amniocentesis was considered a high-risk procedure, and, indeed, for a while the National Institutes of Health declined to support studies that included amniocentesis. Attitudes about the procedure have come around 180 degrees, and the general impression at the moment is that the risk of amniocentesis is trivial. The use of real-time ultrasonography and the performance of these studies in diagnostic centers has significantly reduced the incidence of complications.[1,5,12,13]

In the second trimester the risks consist of infection, abortion, fetal injury, and fetal-maternal transfusion, which can result in isoimmunization of the blood group incompatibility type. One instance of endometriosis of the abdominal wall has also been reported in a woman subjected to three amniocenteses during a single pregnancy for purposes of abortion.[15] Fetal injuries, with second trimester amniocentesis, other than abortion have consisted entirely of small dimples in the fetal skin where the fetus was apparently stuck by the amniocentesis needle. These occurrences were encountered most in the 1960s, prior to the extensive use of ultrasound in guiding the puncture. None has been a serious injury.

The commonest situation in which isoimmunization precipitated by amniocentesis has taken place has been with an Rh-positive fetus in an Rh-negative mother.[14] In approximately 4% of such instances, enough fetal blood gains access to the maternal circulation to create the possibility of sensitization of the mother.[13,20] With abortions performed in the first trimester, the proportion of positive tests for some fetal blood in the mother's blood may be as high as 13%, and in tests near term as high as 26%, but in only a small proportion of these instances is sufficient blood transfused from the fetus into the mother to be responsible for isoimmunization. In any event, it has become standard procedure to administer a prophylactic dose of RhoGAM to the mother when she is Rh negative.[14]

The most serious complication of second trimester amniocentesis has been acknowledged to be abortion. The original summary of this material, published by a group from the U.S. Department of Health, Education, and Welfare, stated that the incidence of abortion among women subjected to amniocentesis was no different from the incidence in controls.[17] Indeed, the publication for the general population distributed by the U.S. Department of Health and Human Services makes a similar statement.[29] However, almost all the large studies, ranging from 1,000 to 3,000 amniocenteses, either in individual institutions or gathered from groups of institutions, have demonstrated a larger incidence of abortion among patients subjected to amniocentesis than among controls.[1,5,12] The collaborative study in Great Britain suggested that this increase was as much as double.[4] Other researchers who have believed that they were studying better control groups and felt more certain of their amniocentesis technique have indicated that the incidence of abortion is much less. However, the incidence of abortion among pregnant women at this period of pregnancy is extremely low, and it would obviously take a very large series to corroborate an increase. It probably can best be approximated at the present time that amniocentesis done in the second trimester, under the best of circumstances, will probably result in less than a 50% increase in the abortion rate. The inherent abortion rate at this duration of pregnancy, however, is certainly not greater than three in a thousand, even in selected high-risk populations of the type that are the subject of amniocentesis.[23]

One thing is certain: The likelihood of complications is directly related to the number of amniocenteses in a particular pregnancy, particularly in the second trimester.[8,15,30]

The complications in the third trimester have a somewhat different configuration. The relative amount of amniotic fluid compared with the fetus, except in instances of polyhydramnios, tends to be much less than it is in the second trimester. As a matter of fact, in severely affected pregnancies with metabolic disorders such as intrauterine growth retardation, one of the features is oligohydramnios, which makes amniocentesis increasingly difficult. Careful ultrasonography to find a safe "window" that gives access to a pool of fluid is of much assistance. Although the risks of rupture of the membranes and induction of premature labor exist in such patients, as well as the risk of amnionitis, the most serious complication, although certainly not the commonest one, is an inadvertent injury to fetal blood vessels. A number of immediate fetal deaths due to hemorrhage from the umbilical cord have been reported. Ordinarily the diagnosis is suggested by the observation of considerable blood in the fluid obtained. This blood can be studied by a rapid screening technique to determine whether or not it is of fetal origin. Because of the severity of this complication, many authors have urged that amniocentesis carried out for diagnostic purposes late in pregnancy be done with continuous monitoring of the fetal heart. In several cases it has been observed that after a bloody tap there was progressive evidence in the fetal monitor of fetal distress, which corroborated the suspicion that the cord had been injured and made it possible to deliver the baby immediately by cesarean section.

A typical instance of this occurred recently in one of my own hospitals. A patient whose prior classical cesarean section warranted abdominal delivery unfortunately had no idea when she conceived. She had presented for care too late to gather critical data. By ultrasound the placenta was seen anteriorly and a presumably safe site for amniocentesis was selected. Upon puncture an initial free flow of clear fluid was followed by gross blood. The baseline fetal heart rate accelerated and then returned to normal while preparation was completed for cesarean delivery. At operation the baby was severely anemic but did well. The placenta and a fetal vessel on its surface had been punctured. Unfortunately, with this complication, not all babies have been salvaged even under the best of circumstances.

The small risk of injuring a fetal vessel must be weighed against the clinical information acquired. As has been mentioned, amniotic fluid need be obtained in only those cases of prior cesarean section where the data are inadequate. In other cases, delivery prior to labor may be mandated by the mother's condition and amniocentesis is therefore unnecessary. In still others, evidence of fetal distress is such that delivery is urgent regardless of findings in the amniotic fluid. In only a small residual group of cases are amniocenteses essential to the clinical decision-making process.

In probably as many as 20% of the cases where amniocentesis is carried out for diagnostic purposes in late pregnancy, there is continuous leak of fluid and premature rupture of membranes, which results in premature delivery.[31] Since almost all these patients are at high risk and are already being considered for premature delivery, it is extremely difficult to measure the clinical impact of this otherwise undesirable accident.

Ethical and Legal Concerns

There are interesting political and legal ramifications of amniocentesis. Fletcher has discussed the ethical issues involved in making determinations of genetic abnormality the basis for abortion.[9] Certainly these issues have arisen in the most dramatic form where one of a pair of twins has been diagnosed as abnormal and procedures are undertaken to kill that fetus with the unpredictable risk of killing a normal co-twin.[16]

Since genetic diagnosis has provided a basis for requests for abortion, the so-called Right-to-Life Movement in the United States has made genetic diagnosis a political target. The National Foundation/March of Dimes for a number of years provided financial support for genetic diagnosis until it fell under severe criticism from the anti-abortion groups. The Muscular Dystrophy Association has experienced similar pressure. Recently, the Utah State Legislature had laid before it legislation to ban all genetic diagnosis except for purposes of intrauterine treatment. It is entirely possible that the human life bill presently before the United States Senate could be interpreted to bar all amniocenteses.

At the other extreme, legal action has been brought against physicians who have failed to urge their patients to undertake genetic diagnosis.[6] The consensus at present is that it is the physician's obligation to recommend amniocentesis to all patients over the age of 35 years, and certainly to all patients with any history of heredofamilial genetic disorders. Since facilities in most genetics laboratories of high quality currently are strained to their limit, these laboratories are in many instances sharply limiting the population to which amniocentesis for diagnosis will be offered.[19,21] This creates new ethical dilemmas. Does a patient have a right to demand that an amniocentesis be done? If we are indeed dedicated to educated consumerism, what response can be made to the patient who at 32 years of age insists that her fear of having an abnormal baby, however uncommon it may be, is so great that she feels that she must have an amniocentesis? If amniocentesis is refused to such a patient, and she subsequently delivers an abnormal child, who can reasonably be expected to bear the immense social cost?

REFERENCES

1. Bartsch F K, Lundberg J, Wahlström J. One thousand consecutive midtrimester amniocenteses. *Obstet Gynecol* 55:305–308, 1980.
2. Birnholz J C, Frigoletto F D. Antenatal treatment of hydrocephalus. *N Engl J Med* 304:1021–1023, 1981.
3. Bowers S K, MacDonald H M, Shapiro E D. Preceding spontaneous labor (PSL), elective repeat cesarean section (RCS), and iatrogenic respiratory distress syndrome (IaRDS). Part 2. *Pediatr Res* 15:652, 1981.
4. Chayen S (ed). An assessment of the hazards of amniocentesis. *Br J Obstet Gynaecol* 85 (suppl 2), 1978.
5. Crandall B F, Howard J, Lebherz T B et al. Follow-up of 2000 second-trimester amniocenteses. *Obstet Gynecol* 56:625–628, 1980.
6. Donovan P. Genetics and the law: Increasing recognition of doctors' duty to warn of foreseeable risks. *Fam Plan Pop Rep* 8(5), 1979.
7. Elias S, et al. Genetic amniocentesis in twin gestations. *Am J Obstet Gynecol* 138:169–173, 1980.
8. Friberg H J, Frigoletto F D. Sonographic demonstration of uterine contraction during amniocentesis. *Am J Obstet Gynecol* 139:740–742, 1981.
9. Fletcher J C. Prenatal diagnosis of the hemoglobinopathies: Ethical issues. *Am J Obstet Gynecol* 135:53–56, 1979.
10. Frigoletto F D, Phillippe M, Davies I J, et al. Avoiding iatrogenic prematurity with elective repeat cesarean section without routine use of amniocentesis. *Am J Obstet Gynecol* 137:521–524, 1980.
11. Garite T J, Freeman R K, Linzey E M, et al. The use of amniocentesis in patients with premature rupture of membranes. *Obstet Gynecol* 54:226–230, 1979.
12. Golbus M S, Loughman W D, Epstein C J, et al. Prenatal genetic diagnosis in 3,000 amniocenteses. *N Engl J Med* 300:157–163, 1979.
13. Harrison R, Campbell S, Craft J. Risks of fetomaternal hemorrhage resulting from amniocentesis with and without ultrasound localization. *Obstet Gynecol* 46:389–391, 1975.
14. Hill L M, Platt L D, Kellogg B. Rh sensitization after genetic amniocentesis. *Obstet Gynecol* 56:459–461, 1980.
15. Kauvitz A, Di Sant'Agnese P A. Needle tract endometriosis: An unusual complication of amniocentesis. *Obstet Gynecol* 54:753–755, 1979.
16. Kerenyi T D, Chitkara U. Selective birth in twin pregnancy with discordancy for Down's syndrome. *N Engl J Med* 304:1525–1527, 1981.

17. Lowe C U, Alexander D, Bryla D, et al. *The safety and accuracy of mid-trimester amniocentesis.* Bethesda, MD, National Institute of Child Health and Human Development, HEW Publication no. 78-190, 1978.

18. Lung problem corrected with baby still in womb. *NY Times* Sept 6, 1981.

19. Marion J P, et al. Acceptance of amniocentesis by low-income patients in an urban hospital. *Am J Obstet Gynecol* 138:11–15, 1980.

20. Mennuti M T, Brummond W, Crombleholme W R, et al. Fetal-maternal bleeding associated with genetic amniocentesis. *Obstet Gynecol* 55:48–54, 1980.

21. Mesirow K H. More on access to amniocentesis. *N Engl J Med* 304:296, 1981.

22. Nolan G H, Schmickel R D, Chantaratherakitti P, et al. The effect of ultrasonography on midtrimester genetic amniocentesis complications. *Am J Obstet Gynecol* 140:531–534, 1981.

23. O'Brien W F. *Assessment of the risks of genetic amniocentesis.* 29th Annual Meeting of Society for Gynecologic Investigation. Mar 24–27, 1982.

24. Pedersen I K, Philip J, Sele V, et al. Monozygotic twins with dissimilar phenotypes and chromosome complements. *Acta Obstet Gynecol Scand* 59:459–462, 1980.

25. Pitkin R. Acute polyhydramnios recurrent in successive pregnancies. *Obstet Gynecol* 48:42S–43S, 1976.

26. Platt L D, Leake R, Sipos L. Amniocentesis in the second trimester: The effect on fetal movement. *Am J Obstet Gynecol* 140:758–759, 1981.

27. Sunder T E. Antenatal treatment of hydrocephalus. *N Engl J Med* 305:403, 1981.

28. Twins born after one undergoes surgery in womb. *NY Times* July 27, 1981.

29. US Department of Health and Human Services: *Amniocentesis for prenatal chromosome diagnosis.* Atlanta, Centers for Disease Control, 1980.

30. Vago T, Chavkin J. Extramembranous pregnancy: An unusual complication of amniocentesis. *Am J Obstet Gynecol* 137:511–512, 1980.

31. Wallace R L, Herrick C N. Amniocentesis in the evaluation of premature labor. *Obstet Gynecol* 57:483–486, 1981.

RECEIVED: SEPTEMBER, 1981
REVISED & ACCEPTED: FEBRUARY, 1982

ULTRASOUND IN CLINICAL OBSTETRICS

David Graham

Since its introduction into obstetrical practice by Ian Donald in the early 1960s, ultrasound has become increasingly utilized for an expanding number of indications. At this time it is difficult to imagine obstetrical practice without the availability of this technology. Since the theory and biological effects of ultrasound are described by Stratmeyer later, the purpose of this chapter is to describe the ways in which ultrasound is utilized in daily clinical practice.

It has been suggested by many that each pregnant woman have at least one sonogram during her pregnancy. There are strong arguments both for and against this approach. The proponents of routine ultrasound suggest that such routine examination would allow detection of otherwise unsuspected multiple pregnancy, fetal growth problems, placental malpositions, and fetal anomalies. Early diagnosis of such conditions would allow earlier intervention and theoretically improve prenatal care. Against such routine uses is the question of availability of facilities and the unanswered questions on long-term safety of ultrasound. At the present time ultrasound facilities are not sufficient to allow routine use in all pregnancies.

Indications for Ultrasound

Although not inclusive, the following are the major indications necessitating an ultrasound examination:

1. For gestational dating, to diagnosis twins, polyhydramnios, or abnormal growth patterns.
2. Assessment of bleeding in pregnancy.
3. Determination of fetal abnormalities.
4. Determination of fetal lie.
5. Guided amniocentesis.
6. Assessment of coexistent mass.

7. Localization of coexistent intrauterine device (IUD).
8. Determination of fetal death.

Normal Pregnancy

At approximately 5 to 6 weeks after the last normal menstrual period, a thin ring of echoes—the gestational sac—representing the trophoblastic shell and the chorionic space may be seen in the uterus. At 6 to 7 weeks gestation a small group of echoes, representing the fetal pole, can be seen within this sac (Fig. 1). Using real-time ultrasound equipment, one can demonstrate fetal movement and fetal heart movement. After 11 to 12 weeks the fetal head is seen as a recognizable structure (Fig. 2), and from this time onward more fetal detail is appreciated as the pregnancy progresses. From about 9 weeks of pregnancy the placenta can be first distinguished. After the first trimester it may be readily seen as a distinct structure (Fig. 3), and its relationship to the internal os, presence of placental anomalies, and degree of placental calcification[6] can be determined.

Ultrasound can show that the relationship of the placenta to the uterus is not fixed but may change as pregnancy advances. This results from a combination of differential growth of the uterus, with the lower segment developing in the last weeks of pregnancy and "growing away" from the placenta, together with technical factors such as the degree of bladder filling.

Assessment of Gestational Age

In the first trimester several methods are available for assessing gestational age: (1) general appearance and presence of certain landmarks, (2) gestational sac diameter, and (3) crown-rump length, which is the longest length of the fetal pole. This measurement correlates extremely well with the gestational age and is probably the most accurate single measurement that can be made in pregnancy (Fig. 1).

After the recognition of the fetal head at about 11 to 12 weeks of gestation the measurement of the biparietal diameter (Fig. 2), a line joining the two parietal bones at their widest distance, is the standard method of assessing gestational age. Up to about 28 to 30 weeks of gestation, growth of the biparietal diameter is linear, the standard deviation being approximately 7 to 11 days.[9] After 28 to 30 weeks the growth of the biparietal diameter slows and the standard deviation becomes wider, so that in the last few weeks of pregnancy the standard deviation of a single examination is approximately 3 weeks.

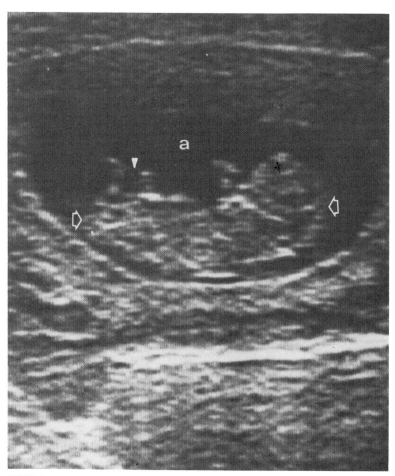

FIGURE 1. Section through gestational sac to show the embryo (open arrows). The fetal head is adjacent to the arrow on the right of the picture. The embryo is surrounded by amniotic fluid (a). Fetal legs may also be seen (closed arrow).

Normal Fetal Anatomy and Fetal Anomalies

From the early part of the second trimester one may visualize fetal anatomy such as intracranial anatomy, cardiac structures, kidneys, bladder, liver, stomach, bowel, and limbs, allowing the diagnosis of certain structural anomalies at a relatively early stage of pregnancy.[7]

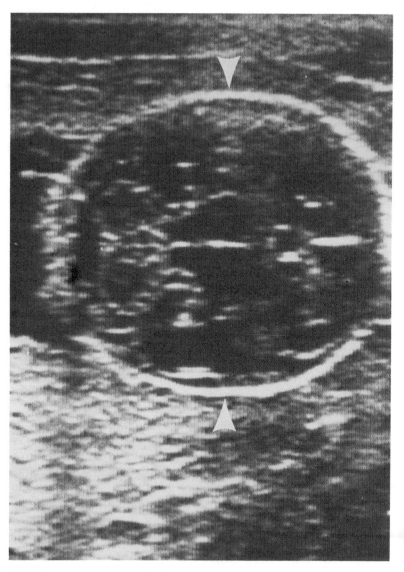

FIGURE 2. Transverse section of fetal head showing fetal cranium at the level used to measure the biparietal diameter (arrows).

Central Nervous System

Current ultrasound equipment allows visualization of intracranial structures such as the ventricles, thalami, cerebral peduncles, and cerebellum. The fetal spine is visualized as two parallel lines in longitudinal view and as a complete circle when seen in transverse view. A number of anomalies of the central nervous system and spine may be diagnosed.[1,7]

1. *Anencephaly.* Failure of closure of the cephalic end of the neural tube may lead to anencephaly, which may be recognized from 13 to 14 weeks gestation by visualization of a small, irregular "nubbin" of tissue representing the base of the skull and facial structures, instead of the normally well-visualized skull and internal structures.

2. *Hydrocephalus.* The lateral ventricles are readily identified on transverse scans of the head. Prior to 17 weeks the ventricles are relatively large in relation to the diameter of the head, but after 17 weeks they should

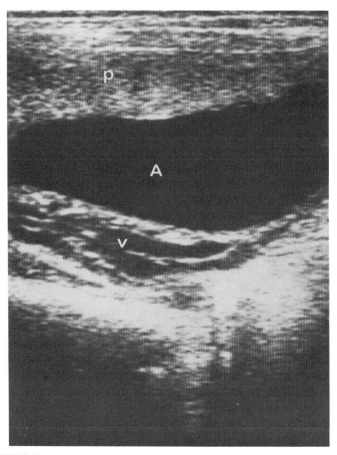

FIGURE 3. Section showing placenta (**p**), amniotic fluid (**A**), and the blood vessels supplying the uterus (**v**). The fetus is not shown.

occupy less than 50% of the diameter of the head.[4] Ventricular dilatation occurs prior to any abnormal increase in head size. Progressive ventricular dilatation and the amount of cortex remaining may be assessed, allowing decisions to be made concerning time of delivery.

3. *Spina bifida*. Spina bifida will be seen as a localized widening of the parallel echoes of the longitudinal view or as a V-shaped or U-shaped spinal canal on the transverse view, rather than the normal complete ring.[1] There may be an associated meningocele visualized as a cystic mass adjacent to the spinal defect. Ultrasound should be utilized along with serum and/or amniotic fluid alpha-fetoprotein estimations to allow detection of those closed defects which might be associated with normal alpha-fetoprotein. Small defects in the lower lumbar and sacral area may be missed on ultrasound examination; however, the alpha-fetoprotein will be elevated in many of these.

4. *Encephalocele*. Encephalocele usually involves the occipital area, and it may be recognized as a cystic mass adjacent to the head that may contain some solid cerebral tissue. The defect in the cranial bone may also be visualized.

5. *Microcephaly*. Microcephaly is most often recognized late in pregnancy. In this condition a consistently smaller biparietal diameter than expected is observed, as well as a discrepancy between the head size and the trunk circumference.

6. Other central nervous system anomalies such as iniencephaly, hydranencephaly, porencephaly, and Dandy-Walker malformations have also been recognized prenatally.

Cardiac Problems

The heart, its component chambers and valve structures, the vena cava, and the aorta are readily recognized with real-time ultrasound (Fig. 4).[8] The heart may be investigated by the following techniques:

1. *M-mode echocardiography*. Using M-mode echocardiography, the clinician may evaluate chamber size, valvular structure and function, and some physiological parameters such as ventricular emptying. Rhythm and conduction disorders may be diagnosed.

2. *Two-dimensional study*. Use of real-time equipment is an extension of the foregoing technique, allowing direct visualization of the cardiac chambers and their function. Congenital anomalies such as ventricular hypoplasia, atrioventricular malformation, and transpositions may be diagnosed.

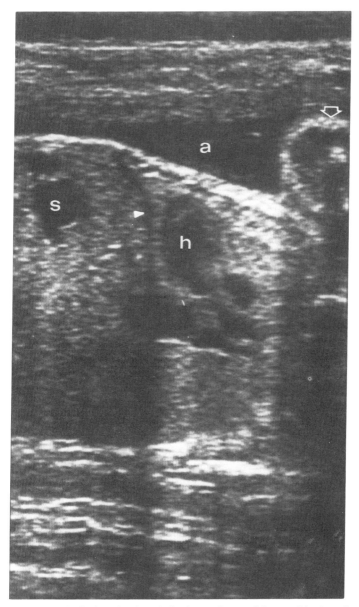

FIGURE 4. Longitudinal section through the chest and upper abdomen of the fetus showing heart (**h**), stomach (**s**), and diaphragm (closed arrow); amniotic fluid is also seen (**a**). A portion of the fetal arm is seen in the upper right (closed arrow).

Pulmonary and Thoracic Problems

Little detail of the lungs is seen in utero. One may visualize the following, however:

1. Pleural effusions, as in fetal hydrops.
2. Cystic adenomatoid malformations of the lung, which usually presents as nonimmune hydrops. Cystic masses may be seen in the chest.
3. Diaphragmatic hernia, in which loops of fluid-filled bowel may be seen in the chest adjacent to the heart.

Gastrointestinal System

Normally the stomach is visualized as a fluid collection in the left upper abdomen. Small segments of bowel are often seen because of their fluid content, especially in later pregnancy. Several gastrointestinal anomalies are diagnosable[7]:

1. Bowel atresias will be visualized as large dilated cystic collections of fluid scattered through the abdomen, the number of loops depending on the level of atresia. Especially with the more proximal atresias, polyhydramnios is often an associated finding.

2. Mesenteric cysts and intestinal duplications may appear as cystic intraabdominal masses.

3. Tracheo-esophageal fistulas are usually associated with polyhydramnios. Although the actual fistula will not be visualized, abnormal swallowing has been described.

4. Omphalocele and gastroschisis are defects involving the anterior abdominal wall. Omphalocele involves a paraumbilical defect, which on ultrasound examination will be shown as an abnormal contour to the abdomen with loops of bowel and/or liver present outside the abdominal cavity. Other structural defects such as cardiac lesions are more common in association with omphalocele. Gastroschisis is a skin-covered paraumbilical defect in the abdominal wall through which intestine eviscerates and is distinguished from omphalocele by its paraumbilical location, normal insertion of the umbilical cord, and lack of an abdominal peritoneal sac containing abdominal viscera.

Skeletal System

Historically, skeletal anomalies have been diagnosed by radiography, often as incidental findings or during study for possible recurrence of a skeletal anatomy. However, with the use of ultrasound one may now diagnose many skeletal problems such as the following, often before such pregnancies are at a stage where radiographic diagnosis is practical[7]:

1. *Dwarfism*. Achondroplasia, thanatophoric dwarfism, and other forms of dwarfism may be diagnosed by finding long-bone lengths (e.g., femur) that are shorter than normal.[5,7]

2. *Osteogenesis imperfecta*. If the fetus is severely affected in utero by the severe variant, fractures of the long bones may occur and be visualized sonographically as bowed, deformed structure. A faint and thin outline to the fetal skull may also be seen.

Genitourinary System

From the early second trimester the fetal kidneys and bladder may be visualized. If sequential scanning is performed over several hours, the bladder may be seen progressively to fill and then empty, and by measuring bladder volumes the urinary production rate may be calculated.

Anomalies of the genitourinary tract may be suspected by the presence of oligohydramnios, where there are bilateral renal anomalies or if there is bladder outlet obstruction.

1. *Hydronephrosis*. Dilatation of the renal pelvis may be visualized by ultrasound and is most often due to a ureteropelvic junction obstruction or, where bilateral, to bladder outlet obstruction. With the latter complication, the bladder will appear as an abnormally large cystic structure in the lower abdomen. Serial sonography will enable assessment of any progressive dilatation of the renal pelvis, allowing a decision to be made concerning whether to continue the pregnancy or to consider early delivery and treatment to prevent further renal damage.

2. *Renal agenesis*. In association with severe oligohydramnios it will be impossible to visualize the renal outlines.

3. *Multicystic kidneys*. Replacement of the normal renal parenchyma by a number of cysts is most often due to multicystic kidney, a renal dysplasia. The affected kidney, or kidneys, is enlarged and when the condition is bilateral, oligohydramnios is usually present.

4. *Infantile polycystic kidney*. Infantile polycystic disease is an autosomal recessive disorder characterized by polycystic kidneys, hepatic fibrosis, and/or pulmonary hypoplasia. With this condition there is enlargement and increased echogenicity of the kidneys and loss of normal corticomedullary differentiation. The cysts are usually too small to be seen separately.

5. *Genital problems*. With careful scanning the external genitalia may be seen in a number of fetuses, allowing sex prediction. In the third trimester, however, the labia occasionally appear prominent and may simulate scrotal appearances. Fetal hydrocele and also ovarian cysts may be diagnosed prenatally, usually as incidental findings.

Soft Tissue Anomalies

1. *Cystic lymphangioma*. This is a congenital malformation of the lymphatic system, the commonest sites being the neck and the axillae. It will be shown as a mass, often cystic in appearance, in the region of the neck. Other soft tissue lesions in this area that are potentially diagnosable are branchial cleft cysts and hemangiomas.

2. *Sacrococcygeal teratoma*. This anomaly has been diagnosed prenatally as a mass in the sacral area protruding from the fetal buttocks.

Miscellaneous Conditions

1. *Fetal hydrops*. The occurrence of fetal pleural effusion, ascites, and skin thickening may be secondary to Rhesus disease or other immune causes, or at the present time more commonly due to nonimmune causes. Nonimmune causes include infections such as cytomegalovirus, renal vein thrombosis, cystic adenomatoid malformation of the lungs, and thalassemia. The ultrasound appearance is characteristic, with pleural and peritoneal fluid collections readily demonstrated.

2. *Diabetes*. In the infant of the diabetic mother, ultrasound may be used to detect abnormal growth patterns such as macrosomia and growth retardation and to detect structural anomalies.

Multiple Pregnancy

Multiple pregnancy can be diagnosed from early in the first trimester when two gestational sacs can be seen. However, there is a significant discrepancy between the number of multiple gestations diagnosed in the first trimester and the number which actually result in twins. It has been estimated that only approximately 30% of twin gestations diagnosed in the first trimester eventually produce twins.[10] This discrepancy is due to a combination of erroneous diagnosis and loss and subsequent resorption of one of the embryos.

When twins are diagnosed after the first trimester, when recognizable fetal anatomy is present, twins are born in the majority of cases.

Ultrasound is of value in the management of twin pregnancy in the following situations:

1. Dating the pregnancy, since the clinical estimation of uterine size will be unreliable;

2. Diagnosis of fetal anomalies that may be more common in twins, especially monochorionic twins;
3. Presence of hydramnios, which when excessive may predispose to premature labor;
4. Evaluation of fetal growth and diagnosis of the twin-to-twin transfusion syndrome. In this latter condition, which may occur in monochorionic twins, one twin receives a disproportionate amount of the placental blood flow and will become plethoric. The "donor" twin will be anemic and growth retarded;
5. Placental position. With the increased size of the placenta, placenta previa will be more common.

Intrauterine Growth Retardation

Using ultrasound, two patterns of intrauterine growth retardation (IUGR) have been described[2]:

1. "Low profile" type, in which the fetus is below average size with a small biparietal diameter throughout the pregnancy. This type of growth retardation is more common with intrauterine infections or congenital anomalies.
2. "Late onset" type, in which fetal biparietal diameter measurements are normal until approximately 28 to 30 weeks, when there will be seen slowing of the incremental growth of the biparietal diameter. This type of growth retardation is more common in placental insufficiency (e.g., in hypertension or diabetes).

As well as the biparietal diameter, other parameters that can be used in suspected IUGR are the total intrauterine volume (TIUV), which is decreased in IUGR, and the ratio of head circumference to the circumference of the trunk, measured at the umbilical vein. The head-to-trunk ratio will be normal in the symmetrical type of IUGR ("low profile") and increased in asymmetrical ("late onset") IUGR.

Fetal Well-Being

Several techniques are available to assess the well-being of the fetus. Methods most commonly used at the present time are fetal heart rate monitoring using Doppler ultrasound (the nonstress test) and measurement of the estrogen metabolite estriol in a 24-hour urine collection. When normal, both of these investigations are reassuring of satisfactory fetoplacental function. More recently, ultrasound evaluation of several physiological parameters including fetal breathing, tone, and movement have been proposed as an additional method of assessing fetal well-being.[11] These parameters, together with estimation of oligohydramnios and the nonstress test, have been combined to form a "planning score." A high score is reassuring of normal fetoplacental function—and a low score prior to delivery is associated with a high perinatal morbidity and mortality.

Bleeding in Early Pregnancy

Vaginal bleeding occurs in about 25% of all early pregnancies. When local lesions have been excluded and the cervix is closed, ultrasound should be employed to determine fetal viability. Using ultrasound, the pregnancy may be placed in one of the following categories:

1. Appearances are normal and appropriate to the gestational age. These patients are more likely to progress to term, although bleeding may recur.

2. "Blighted ovum" or anembryonic pregnancy. A poorly defined gestational sac, smaller than expected and not containing a fetal pole, may be seen. In the appropriate clinical situation, the ultrasound appearances are usually characteristic. If, however, there is doubt about the appearances, a repeat examination in 10 to 14 days will distinguish between a very early normal pregnancy, which will show appropriate interval growth, and the blighted ovum, which will show little or no growth.

3. Missed abortion. Where the fetus has died some weeks prior to the bleeding episode, ultrasound may show a uterus that is much smaller than expected for the time of amenorrhea and that may contain an immobile fetal pole or no recognizable fetal structures.

Bleeding in Late Pregnancy

In the patient presenting with bleeding in the third trimester of pregnancy, the main diagnostic considerations are placenta previa, where a portion of the placenta covers the internal os, or placental abruption, a premature separation of a portion of the placenta. Since clinical management of the two conditions is completely different, ultrasound is used as an initial investigation to determine the placental position in relation to the internal os. Since the appearance of the lower segment may change when the bladder is distended, the patient in whom placenta previa is diagnosed when the bladder is full should be rescanned when the bladder is empty to determine whether the appearances are persistent. Because of the possibility of change in placental position with advancing gestation, the diagnosis of placenta previa should be confirmed by rescanning prior to any decision being made concerning the mode of delivery. Occasionally, blood from the placenta previa will collect in front of the internal os and be visualized sonographically.

Abruption is more difficult to diagnose definitively with ultrasound and is usually diagnosed after placenta previa and local causes have been excluded. In a situation where there has been major separation of the placenta with a large retroplacental clot, the ultrasound appearances are often striking with visible detachment of the placenta and a heterogeneous collection of echoes behind the placenta due to clotted blood. Lesser degrees of abruption may show no definite changes on ultrasound—occasionally one may see a definite retroplacental collection or partial separation. Occasionally, blood tracking down to the lower uterus may collect in the area of the internal os and be visualized—it may, in fact, mimic placenta previa. In normal pregnancy often there is a wide area of lucency inferior to the placenta, representing blood vessels that may mimic placental separation and be misdiagnosed as such.

Fetal Death in Utero

With real-time ultrasound, fetal movement and fetal cardiac activity are usually readily appreciated. Absence of fetal cardiac movement where the fetal heart is seen is indicative of fetal death. In situations where fetal death has occurred several days prior to the examination, secondary nonspecific changes may be seen, including overlapping of cranial bones, unusual fetal positions, and thickening of the scalp echoes.

Amniocentesis

Amniocentesis is sampling of the amniotic fluid by transabdominal passage of a needle. There are several indicators for amniocentesis, as follows:

1. *Midtrimester or genetic amniocentesis.* Amniocentesis is performed at approximately 16 to 17 weeks of gestation and fluid analyzed for the following:

a. *Fetal cells.* Fetal fibroblasts are grown in culture and karyotyped to diagnose chromosomal anomalies (e.g., Down's syndrome).

b. *Estimation of alpha-fetoprotein (AFP).* AFP is a protein synthesized by the fetus that normally may be detected in the amniotic fluid and in maternal serum. Abnormally elevated AFP may be found in certain fetal conditions, such as neural tube defect, tracheo-esophageal fistula, duodenal atresia, and congenital nephrosis.

c. *Determination of enzyme activity in fetal cells or amniotic fluid.* Approximately 75 autosomal recessive conditions manifested by enzyme deficiencies can be diagnosed in such a manner, for example, Tay-Sachs disease, a condition especially common in Ashkenazi Jews, in which affected fetuses have low levels of the enzyme hexosaminidase A.

In midtrimester amniocentesis, ultrasound is of value in the following situations:

a. Choice of a suitable location of needle insertion, avoiding the placenta where possible, avoiding the fetus and umbilical cord, and decreasing the number of bloody or unsuccessful taps.[3]

b. Determination of gestational age. To allow correction of AFP levels and to determine the optimal time for amniocentesis.

c. Diagnosis of multiple pregnancy. When twins are present, both sacs may be aspirated under ultrasound guidance.

d. Diagnosis of fetal death.

e. Diagnosis of certain congenital anomalies.

f. Diagnosis of coexistent masses that may interfere with amniocentesis.

2. *Third trimester amniocentesis.* In the third trimester, amniocentesis ultrasound is again of great value in determining the optimal site for needle insertion, avoiding placenta, umbilical cord, and vital fetal structures and therefore decreasing the complications of this procedure.

Coexistent Masses in Pregnancy

With ultrasound, adnexal masses detected on pelvic examination may be characterized as to their nature, that is, solid or cystic, unilocular or multilocular. A unilocular cystic mass found in association with a first trimester pregnancy most commonly is a corpus luteum cyst, and detection may be followed by clinical examination or ultrasound. A mass that is shown by ultrasound to be multilocular or having a significant amount of solid tissue is unlikely to be a corpus luteum cyst and should be managed accordingly.

Fibroids are not uncommonly associated with pregnancy, especially in the older woman and, when large, may distort the uterine cavity and predispose to infertility or spontaneous abortion. When the pregnancy progresses into the third trimester, there is a higher incidence of premature rupture of membranes, premature labor, antepartum bleeding, and postpartum bleeding. Fibroids in pregnancy may be detected sonographically by a localized abnormality in the uterine contour or by an area of changed echo texture.

Localization of Intrauterine Device (IUD)

Where the string of the device is not seen and the patient is pregnant, ultrasound will allow localization of the IUD and its relationship to the gestational sac. An extrauterine IUD may be impossible to visualize, since it may lie between loops of bowel that prevent passage of the ultrasound.

Pelvimetry

Although ultrasound has been advocated as a means of assessing various parameters of the pelvis, this has not become a routine procedure because of the limited information obtained and technical difficulty.

REFERENCES

1. Campbell S. Early prenatal diagnosis of neural tube defects by ultrasound. *Clin Obstet Gynecol* 20:351–359, 1977.

2. Campbell S, Thoms A. Ultrasound measurement of the fetal head to abdomen circumference ratio in the assessment of growth retardation. *Br J Obstet Gynaecol* 84:165–174, 1977.

3. Chandra P, Nitowsky HM, Marion R, et al. Experience with sonography as an adjunct to amniocentesis for prenatal diagnosis of fetal genetic disorders. *Am J Obstet Gynecol* 133:519–524, 1979.

4. Renkhaus M, Winsberg F. Ultrasonic measurement of the fetal ventricular system. *Radiology* 131:781–787, 1979.

5. Filly RA, Golbus MS, Carey JC, et al. Short limbed dwarfism: Ultrasonic diagnosis by mensuration of fetal femoral length. *Radiology* 138:653–656, 1981.

6. Grannum PA, Berkowitz RL, and Hobbins JC: The ultrasonic changes in the maturing placenta and their relation to fetal pulmonic maturity. *Am J Obstet Gynecol* 133:915–922, 1976.

7. Hobbins J C, Grannum P A, Berkowitz R L, et al. Ultrasound in the diagnosis of congenital anomalies. *Am J Obstet Gynecol* 134:331–345, 1979.

8. Kleinman C S, Hobbins J C, Jaffe C C, et al. Echocardiographic studies of the human fetus: Prenatal diagnosis of congenital heart disease and cardiac dysrhythmias, *Pediatrics* 65:1059–1066, 1980.

9. Kurz B A, Wapner R J, Jurtz R J, et al. Analysis of biparietal diameter as an accurate indicator of gestational age. *J Clin Ultrasound* 8:319–326, 1980.

10. Levi S. Ultrasonic assessment of the high rate of human multiple pregnancy in the first trimester. *J Clin Ultrasound* 4:3–5, 1976.

11. Manning, F A, Platt, L D. Antepartum fetal evaluation, development of a fetal biophysical profile. *Am J Obstet Gynecol* 136:787, 1980.

12. Pystynen P, Ylostalo P, Jarvinen P. Pelvimetry by ultrasound in late pregnancy. *Ann Chir Gynaecol Fenn* 56:118–21, 1967.

13. Queenan J T, O'Brien G D, Campbell S. Ultrasound measurement of fetal limb bones. *Am J Obstet Gynecol* 138:297–302, 1980.

14. Robinson H P, Fleming J E. A critical evaluation of sonar "crown-rump length" measurements. *Br J Obstet Gynaecol* 82:702–710, 1975.

RECEIVED: APRIL, 1981
REVISED & ACCEPTED: JUNE, 1981

DIAGNOSTIC ULTRASOUND IN OBSTETRICS AND GYNECOLOGY*

Because of its unique diagnostic capability, relative safety, and noninvasiveness, ultrasound has assumed an important role in obstetrics and gynecology. Ultrasound can provide valuable supplemental information, but it cannot be a substitute for a careful history, physical examination, and sound clinical judgment.

Availability

Since diagnostic ultrasound is an integral part of obstetrics and gynecology, it should be available on a 24-hour basis in all hospitals designated as secondary and tertiary perinatal care centers. Although every hospital may not have equipment available on the premises, for optimum patient care, ultrasound should be accessible within the area.

Ultrasound Operators

The degree of knowledge and skill of the operator is more a important consideration than the orientation of basic training, whether it be in obstetrics and gynecology or in radiology. It is now relatively easy to gain access to ultrasound, but the use of this technique without proper training could result in false diagnoses and reduced cost-effectiveness.

Only a small percentage of physicians have adequate formal training in the use of ultrasound. Ideally, a physician should train at a medical center, learning ultrasound by performing procedures under the guidance of experimental professionals. Further training may be gained from postgraduate courses. The addition of ultrasonography instruction to the curriculum of residency programs in obstetrics and gynecology and radiology will lessen the problem of physician training in the future, but the rapidly changing technology makes continuing education necessary and increasingly important.

*ACOG Technical Bulletin Number 63, October, 1981. Reprinted with permission from The American College of Obstetricians and Gynecologists, 600 Maryland Avenue, SW, Washington, DC.

Ultrasound technologists should complete accredited training programs and qualify for certification by the American Society of Ultrasound Technical Specialists (ASUTS). In all instances technicians should work under the direct supervision of physicians knowledgeable in ultrasound.

Each time a patient undergoes a diagnostic scan, representative photographs or reproductions of that examination should be retained and a report of the findings of the procedure should be recorded. This report should be signed by the individual responsible for the diagnostic ultrasound service.

Instrumentation

The ultrasound image may be altered by increasing or decreasing the gain control. It is important that each laboratory know the capabilities of their equipment and adjust the gain controls daily in relation to the full urinary bladder to achieve a clear delineation between cystic and solid structures.

New technology offers continual improvements in resolution that will enable the clinician to identify smaller structures and minute tissue density changes. The majority types of diagnostic equipment commonly used are static B-scan, real-time imaging, and Doppler ultrasound.

Static B-scan or pulsed ultrasound, allows the clinician to obtain a 2-dimensional, cross-sectional image of anatomical structures. Repeated scans are performed in both a longitudinal and transverse plan in order to obtain a composite display.

Real-time imaging displays moving structures. The image of anatomical structures is similar to that of a motion picture. Real-time ultrasound is particularly valuable for viewing fetal and cardiac activity.

Doppler ultrasound employs a two-crystal transducer that continuously emits and receives sound waves. Echoes returning from moving structures are recorded as audio signals. In obstetrics, Doppler ultrasound is used for fetal heart rate monitoring.

Safety

Ultrasound instruments do not emit ionizing radiation. Energy is produced in the form of sound waves, which are directed through the body and reflect off the structure being imaged. The intensity of the waves may vary from a very high intensity, as in diathermy, to the very low intensity used in diagnostic instruments.

The intensity of energy waves emitted from an instrument is measured in milliwatts/centimeter at the face of the transducer. The level at the object being imaged will be less because of the dispersement of energy in tissue. With the new focused transducers the energy is measured at spacial peak. Commercially available diagnostic instruments emit 5–20 mW/cm² (0.005–0.020 W/cm²). Tissue damage has been reported with energy emissions in the area of 1000 W/cm². No tissue damage has been shown with the emission of energy levels from 5–20 mW/cm² (0.005–0.020 W/cm²).

Diagnostic B-scan ultrasound instruments emit a *pulsed* sound wave. Doppler fetal heart rate detectors utilize *continuous* wave ultrasound. It is difficult to assess which method exposes the patient to more energy. The *continuous* wave technique employs two crystals, one for emitting a continuous sound wave and another for receiving the sound wave, operating at a low energy peak. The *pulsed* wave method employs one crystal that emits sound waves and then receives its echoes. The duration the crystal is emitting sound waves is a small fraction of the time the crystal is receiving the echoes, but this method requires a higher peak energy than continuous wave ultrasound.

All commercially available ultrasound equipment (emitting 5–20 mW/cm²) appears to be safe from the standpoint of the mother and fetus. However, ultrasound should be used judiciously and only when indicated.

Ultrasound in Obstetrics

Ultrasound has a broader application to obstetrics than to gynecology. Listed below are the primary indications for its use:

1. Gestational age
   A. Gestational sac diameter (average): 5–8 weeks
   B. Crown rump length: 8–14 weeks
   C. Biparietal diameter (BPD): 15–25 weeks
2. Abnormalities of early pregnancy
   A. Hydatidiform mole
   B. Ectopic pregnancy
   C. Threatened or missed abortion
   D. Congenital malformations, fetal and maternal
3. Pre- and post-amniocentesis studies
   A. Placental localization
   B. Second trimester amniocentesis
   C. Third trimester amniocentesis
   D. Fetal motion

4. Fetal growth studies (BPD, second trimester)
   A. Normal
   B. Retarded
   C. Accelerated
5. Vaginal bleeding
   A. Missed abortion
   B. Placenta previa
   C. Ectopic pregnancy
   D. Hydatidiform mole
   E. Abruptio placentae
6. Presentation of fetus
7. Multiple pregnancies
8. Congenital malformations
9. Fetal life (extremity and cardiac motion)
10. Pelvic masses

Scanning

Adequate scanning. When caring for a patient, clinical situations often arise that make it more appropriate to order an initial general examination rather than a specific ultrasound procedure. For instance, if a fetal biparietal diameter (BPD) is requested, some services provide only the requested information without performing a complete evaluation of the pregnancy and the pelvis. When assuming responsibility for scanning a patient, the sonographer should perform a complete examination. An error of omission could seriously jeopardize a patient's care. An initial scan should include evaluation and recording of: The number of gestational sacs or fetuses, including presentation, gestational age, and presence of motion or congenital malformations; the location and features of the placenta; an estimation of amniotic fluid volume; and the presence of any abnormal pelvic masses.

Routine versus indicated scans. Third party payors have recently refused to pay for routine screening procedures. No well-controlled study has yet proved that routine scanning of all prenatal patients will improve the outcome of pregnancy. Furthermore, it is possible for information obtained from routine ultrasound scanning to be misinterpreted, which could mislead the clinician.

If routine scanning of all prenatal patients were performed at 20–24 weeks' gestation, the incidence of abnormal presentations and apparent placenta previa would far exceed the actual occurrence at term. At 20–24 weeks' gestation abnormal presentations occur in 35% of patients. The incidence at term is 4%. At 20–24 weeks' gestation, the placenta appears to be low lying or placenta previa in more than 20% of patients. The incidence of placenta previa at term is 0.5%. Therefore, routine screening with ultrasound could indicate an incidence of abnormal presentations that appears to be nine times the real occurrence at term. The apparent incidence of placenta previa could be 60 times the actual occurrence at term. Some of the major and many of the minor congenital malformations would be missed, thus the apparent incidence of congenital malformations would be less than the real occurrence at term. At the present, only indicated diagnostic studies should be ordered.

Pitfalls in Ultrasound Diagnosis

Multiple pregnancies. The ultrasound scan images in only one plane at a time; therefore, it is theoretically possible to overlook the presence of an additional fetus. Real-time imaging is particularly suited to diagnose multiple pregnancy and should be accurate. If there is doubt, the ultrasound scan should be repeated in 2–3 weeks. If the ultrasonic interpretation is still uncertain, a static ultrasound examination should be performed. A roentgenogram should not be needed for multiple fetal diagnosis.

Fetal biparietal diameter. Measurement of the fetal BPD is the most commonly used method for determining gestational age. The fetal BPD correlates most accurately with gestational age between 15–25 weeks' gestation (plus or minus 10 days); after that time the correlation decreases to within plus or minus 3 weeks' gestation.

In order to obtain an accurate BPD, a proper image of the fetal head showing the largest BPD should be displayed. When the correct plane is found, the head will appear round or slightly ovoid with a distinct midline echo. The thalami should be visible. The widest transverse measurement is determined as the BPD. Scans should be repeated until three consistent measurements are obtained.

When the head is in the occiput anterior or occiput posterior position or deep in the pelvis, failure to properly image the head occurs in 5% of cases. In these positions, the ultrasound beam cannot be directed perpendicular to the falx cerebri because of the maternal iliac bones.

The earlier in pregnancy a BPD is determined, the more precise it will be as an estimation of gestational age. Since a single BPD measurement obtained late in pregnancy (beyond 25 weeks' gestation) is accurate only within plus or minus 3 weeks, it is important to realize that a BPD determination at 38 weeks' gestation to determine fetal maturity for induction of labor can be misleading. A mean value for 38 weeks' gestation can represent an actual 38-week gestation or a large-for-dates 35-week fetus.

Although BPD measurements vary from one population to another, it is acceptable to use the values supplied from a nearby medical center or the composite mean values shown in Table 1. Although it may take a long time to achieve, ultimately each laboratory should develop specific values for its patients.

Intrauterine growth retardation. Fetal growth can be determined by a number of ultrasonographic methods. It is extremely important that the ultrasonographer examine the fetus over a sufficient time span to be certain that fetal growth is truly retarded. If BPD measurements are used for determination of intrauterine growth retardation (IUGR), it should be remembered that establishment of accurate dates of pregnancy is essential for interpretation of BPD values. A BPD determination must be obtained in the early second trimester for accurate dating of pregnancy. Most accurate methods presently available include total intrauterine volume measurements, which cannot be performed with real-time equipment. Since determination of inadequate fetal growth depends upon somewhat sophisticated measurement of fetal dimensions, it may be advantageous to consider a consultation with a perinatal center to avoid the grave consequences of a false positive or a false negative diagnosis. Other methods of evaluating IUGR include head/abdomen ratios, head/thorax ratios, and total intrauterine volume determination.

Placenta previa. Ultrasound is particularly valuable in determining placental location. It is, therefore, extremely useful in assessing second and third trimester bleeding. In mid-pregnancy, however, it must be remembered that the placenta appears to be implanted low or covering the cervical os in 30–40% of patients.

Since the actual incidence of placenta previa at term is 0.5%, many apparent cases of placenta previa are not clinically significant in early pregnancy. The term *migrating placenta* has been used to describe the placenta that is observed in close approximation to the cervix at mid-pregnancy but that appears in the fundus at term. Obviously, the placenta does not migrate, but since the uterus grows rapidly in the course of a pregnancy and the lower uterine segment develops by term, a change in the position of the placenta relative to the lower uterine section occurs. A tentative diagnosis of placenta previa early in pregnancy must be always followed up with ultrasound scanning near term, if clinically indicated, to determine if it remains a problem at the time of delivery.

Congenital malformation. With the rapid evolution of the field of genetics there is an increasing indication for the use of ultrasound in detecting congenital malformation syndromes. A variety of congenital malformations in-

TABLE 1.   Composite mean values of BPD

Weeks' gestation	Composite mean (cm)
14	2.8
15	3.2
16	3.6
17	3.9
18	4.2
19	4.5
20	4.8
21	5.1
22	5.4
23	5.8
24	6.1
25	6.4
26	6.7
27	7.0
28	7.2
29	7.5
30	7.8
31	8.0
32	8.2
33	8.5
34	8.7
35	8.8
36	9.0
37	9.2
38	9.3
39	9.4
40	9.5

Sabbagha RE, Hughey M: Standardization of sonar cephalometry and gestational age. Obstet Gynecol 52:402, 1978

volving the head, spine, chest, abdomen, and extremities can be diagnosed with ultrasound. Diagnosis of the following congenital malformations have been reported: Hydrocephaly, anencephaly, spina bifida, meningocele, intrathoracic cysts, cardiac defects, gastrointestinal obstructions, genitourinary strictures, renal dysplasia, and skeletal dysplasias. Most of these diagnoses are difficult to make and require experience with specialized techniques.

The diagnosis of major abnormalities of the fetal head, such as hydrocephaly, anencephaly, and microcephaly may be made with relative certainty. Anytime a BPD is obtained, the lateral ventricular size should be assessed. Detecting a spina bifida or meningocele, however, is more difficult, especially when they occur in the cervical or lower lumbar area.

Ultrasound in Gynecology

With the technological advances in gray scale imaging and the refined ability to differentiate tissue densities, the use of ultrasound in gynecology is rapidly increasing. In most instances it is confined to confirmation of an already suspected clinical problem. The value of ultrasound is in determining the characteristics of a mass: cystic versus solid; adnexal versus uterine; structure (i.e., loculated or simple); describing its shape (i.e., smooth or irregular); measuring its exact size; and evaluating intrauterine contents (i.e., pregnancy, intrauterine contraceptive device).

Meticulous scanning techniques and appreciation of pelvic anatomy are of the utmost importance in evaluation of the pelvis. Because of the small field of view with a real-time system, most gynecologic examinations are usually done with the static system. The technician must be alert to detect unsuspected findings. A pelvic examination during a real-time scan may give additional information concerning pelvic lesions.

The clinical problems in which diagnostic ultrasound is helpful are simple ovarian cysts, tubo-ovarian abscess, hydatidiform mole, extrauterine pregnancy, dermoid cyst, ascites, and location of an intrauterine contraceptive device. Ultrasound can also be useful for patients with myomata or ovarian tumors to assess tumor response to therapy.

Conclusion

Ultrasound has proven to be a valuable asset in the practice of obstetrics and gynecology, and its use will continue to increase as improved technology becomes available. The rapidly changing nature of the field requires constant updating of clinical information through independent research and review as new advances are made in the future.

REFERENCES

Campbell S: Ultrasonic fetal cephalometry during the second trimester of pregnancy. *J Obstet Gynaecol Br Commonw* 77:1057, 1970

Hellman LM, Kobayashi M, Fillisti L, et al: Growth and development of the human fetus prior to the twentieth week of gestation. *Am J Obstet Gynecol* 103:789, 1969

Hobbins JC, et al: Ultrasound in the diagnosis of congenital anomalies. *Am J Obstet Gynecol* 134:3, 1979

Hobbins JC, Berkowitz RL, Hohler CW: How safe is ultrasound in obstetrics? *Contemp Ob/Gyn* 14:63, 1980

Robinson HP: Sonar measurement of fetal crown-rump length as means of assessing maturity in first trimester of pregnancy. *Br Med J* 4:28, 1973

Sabbagha RE, Hughey M: Standardization of sonar cephalometry and gestational age. *Obstet Gynecol* 52:402, 1978

This Technical Bulletin is prepared by the Committee on Technical Bulletins of The American College of Obstetricians and Gynecologists. The Committee wishes to thank John T. Queenan, M.D., FACOG, for assistance in authoring the text. It describes methods and techniques of clinical practice that are currently acceptable and used by recognized authorities. However, it does not represent official policy or recommendations of The American College of Obstetricians and Gynecologists. Its publication should not be construed as excluding other acceptable methods of handling similar problems.

BIOLOGICAL EFFECTS OF ULTRASOUND

Melvin E. Stratmeyer
Christopher L. Christman

Ultrasound is a mechanical vibration (sound) at frequencies above the normal level of human hearing (20 kHz or 20,000 cycles per second). It is a nonionizing form of radiation that is used in diagnostic medicine to visualize soft tissue structure (pulse-echo techniques) and to detect movement within the body such as monitoring the fetal heart during pregnancy and delivery (Doppler techniques). At present the diagnostic use of ultrasound is accepted as safe. This acceptance is based on animal experiments that show an apparent threshold below which effects observed at high levels of exposure do not occur. Acceptance is reinforced by the apparent absence of reports of acute adverse effects in humans. Before examining the available evidence of ultrasound-induced effects in humans and laboratory systems to determine if this acceptance of safety is justified, a brief discussion of possible acoustic mechanisms of interaction with tissue is included to aid in evaluating the evidence.

Mechanisms

When studying harmful effects, there are at least two ways to quantify an ultrasonic interaction with tissue: by specifying the strength of the exposure field or by specifying the acoustic energy absorbed by the tissue. The choice of the better one to use as an index of risk depends on the mechanism causing the observed biological effect. Three mechanisms have been identified that could cause biological damage. They are sonically generated heat, cavitation, and radiation force.[1,2] Because two of these mechanisms, cavitation and radiation force, do not necessarily depend on a tissue temperature rise, whereas the other mechanism clearly does, both thermal and nonthermal mechanisms must be considered when investigating ultrasonically induced biological effects.

When a plane wave propagates through a homogeneous medium, its intensity is decreased by an amount that depends on the absorption coefficient of the medium. This loss of sonic energy is converted into heat, which causes a localized temperature rise. Although the heat transfer process in biological tissues is extremely complex because the circulation system tends to thermally regulate the animal, there is a critical temperature which, if exceeded, causes irreversible damage to the tissue. Therefore, when assessing the risk of ultrasonic exposure to thermal damage, the absorption coefficients of the appropriate tissues must be known. Although a vast amount of data have been accumulated about the acoustic properties of various mammalian tissues,[3,4] most of these data give attenuation coefficients, which include energy scattered by inhomogeneities in the tissue as well as energy absorbed by the tissue. Therefore care should be exercised when using these data.

Absorption is normally considered to be linear and thus independent of acoustic intensity. For high intensities, this assumption is no longer valid when the initial sinusoidal waveform becomes distorted and is converted into a shock wave that resembles a sawtooth pattern. One consequence of shock formation is an increase in the rate at which sonic energy is converted into heat. This phenomenon is called nonlinearly induced absorption and is only one of several physical observations that have been collectively referred to as finite-wave effects. Their importance in biomedical applications has been discussed elsewhere.[5] Although it appears that current diagnostic devices used for visualization produce peak intensities high enough to cause shock formation in water,[6] the possibility of shock formation in tissue is still unknown and requires further study.

Cavitation is another mechanism used to explain biological effects that have been observed after ultrasound exposure. This phenomenon has been subdivided theoretically into a stable and transient form.[7] Stable cavitation describes the interaction between a sound field and a gas-filled bubble, in which the bubble's surface oscillates radially in response to local pressure variations caused by the acoustic wave. Whenever a bubble oscillates, energy is extracted in the form of heat and re-radiated spherical waves. The magnitude of these oscillations reaches a maximum for the bubble's resonant size and may produce large local stresses and elevated temperatures. During stable cavitation, bubble oscillations persist for at least several acoustic cycles and may last indefinitely. Transient cavitation, on the other hand, describes the violent collapse of a gas bubble during the negative portion of a single acoustic cycle. For transient cavitation, temperatures high enough to dissociate water molecules into free radicals can be generated.

An essential ingredient for the inception of cavitation is the existence of gas-filled cavities, or micronuclei. These cavities can form *de novo* during ultrasound exposures, but only when acoustic pressures are extremely high.[8] Because such high intensities are unlikely during the medical use of ultrasound, cavitation events in tissue depend on the presence of micronuclei *in vivo*. To be biologically important, these micronuclei must also be near resonant size. If smaller, they may grow to resonant size during ultrasound exposure by a process called rectified diffusion.[9] This process is relatively slow and probably would not be significant for microsecond pulses that are now typical of commercial pulse-echo scanners.

Certain biological systems have been chosen for experimentation because they are known to contain gas pockets. For example, bean roots have been used to investigate cavitation because, like many plant tissues, they contain intercellular spaces filled with gas.[10] Fruit flies (*Drosophila melanogaster*) also have been used as experimental specimens because the respiratory system of insects may provide tissue with a stable distribution of gas bodies that are near resonant size at megahertz frequencies.[11] Although micronuclei do exist in some biological systems, their existence in mammalian tissue has not been conclusively established. Harvey's experiments with resting cats and dogs suggest that some micronuclei are normally present in mammals which cause profuse bubble formation during decompression.[12] Additional evidence for the existence of micronuclei in mammalian tissue comes from a report of bubble formation in the hind limbs of guinea-pigs exposed to therapeutic levels of ultrasound.[13] The size distribution of *in vivo* micronuclei is unknown and may not fall within the critical range necessary to produce cavitation during the clinical use of ultrasound.

Mechanical effects are another mechanism that can lead to biological damage during ultrasound exposure. Using basic nonlinear equations of acoustics, Nyborg has shown that the acoustic velocity contains a static term which represents a time independent fluid flow called microstreaming.[14] Because of high velocity gradients and the corresponding large shear stresses that are sometimes produced, this phenomenon has been implicated as a possible mechanism to explain the hemolysis of red blood cells.[15] A static term for the acoustic pressure also occurs that represents a radiation force. Such forces may produce sonically generated torques that cause intracellular bodies to rotate when a cell boundary is set into vibration. For standing wave exposure fields, the radiation force will be periodic in half-wavelength intervals. In a comprehensive analysis of blood cell banding in chick embryos, ter Haar concludes that standing wave radiation pressure forces are responsible for the positions of the bands.[16]

Dosimetry

The problem of how to relate a physical variable associated with the ultrasonic field to a biologically significant change is not unique for ultrasound exposures but is common to all forms of radiation. The study of such problems is collectively referred to as dosimetry. O'Brien has traced the development of dosimetric principles in ionizing research and has discussed their use for ultrasound biological effect studies.[17] He points out that the particular dosimetric quantity which will be most useful for an investigation depends on the mechanism of interaction. If temperature rise produces the observed effect, the amount and rate of ultrasonic energy absorbed per unit mass will be important. If cavitation is the mechanism producing the effect, the internal acoustic pressure may be a more useful quantity to measure.

Most biological effect experiments conducted to date have specified exposure conditions less rigorously. This is usually done by measuring the free-field spatial average intensity at the face of the transducer, a quantity given by the total acoustic output power from the source divided by its active radiating area. Although spatial average intensity is convenient to measure, it does not adequately account for the complexity of the exposure field. To account for spatial variations, the peak acoustic intensity in a plane parallel to the transducer is sometimes specified. Spatial peak to spatial average intensity ratios are usually between 2 and 6 for unfocused transducers and will decrease as the distance from the transducer is increased. For focused transducers this ratio may be much higher.

To account for temporal variations that occur during pulse exposures, additional dosimetric quantities must be specified. The temporal peak intensity is the maximum value of the instantaneous intensity that occurs during the pulse burst, whereas the temporal average intensity is the time average of the instantaneous intensity, averaged over one or more pulse periods. Because of short pulse lengths and relatively low pulse repetition rates, temporal peak intensities for pulse-echo scanners are typically three orders of magnitude greater than their temporal average intensities. For simplicity, dosimetric terms presented here have not been defined rigorously. Interested readers are urged to consult the American Institute of Ultrasound in Medicine Standards Committee recommended nomenclature for more complete definitions.[18]

Continuous wave diagnostic ultrasound devices used in obstetrics generally employ frequencies of approximately 2 MHz and output intensities ranging from less than 1 to 20 mW/cm². Pulsed ultrasound devices used in obstetrics generally employ frequencies in the 1 to 10 MHz range with spatial average, temporal average output intensities ranging from less than 1 to 10 mW/cm². However, the temporal peak output intensities of pulsed ultrasound devices are in the W/cm² range.[19]

Although quantifying the exposure field in terms of intensity parameters is useful, the complexity of the exposure field changes with distance from the transducer and makes it difficult to compare results for different exposure protocols when attempting a risk assessment analysis. This problem is further complicated because the acoustic field, usually measured without the biological specimen, is expected to change when the specimen is included. To overcome some of these difficulties, work has been done to quantify internal dosimetric parameters.[20] Although new dosimetric techniques are constantly being developed, the bulk of existing biological effect data were taken under conditions in which there is uncertainty in internal dosimetric parameters. Therefore, any threshold based on the following biological evidence for ultrasound-induced effects must be considered to be only an order-of-magnitude estimate.

Human Studies

Table 1 lists the human studies known to have been conducted on the biological effects of diagnostic ultrasound as it is used in obstetrics. Only two studies have reported positive results. The first reported an increase in chromosome breaks in cultured fetal cells from amniotic fluid exposed *in vivo*.[25] Although the investigators considered the damage to be pathological at the time, the results were not statistically significant nor confirmed by other investigators. The second report involved a study of the effect of Doppler ultrasound on fetal activity. In this study a significant increase in fetal activity was observed in patients exposed to ultrasound compared to sham exposed patients;[29] however, in another study done under similar conditions, no increase in fetal activity was observed.[30] Although most of the human studies failed to show a relationship between the endpoint being studied and fetal exposure to ultrasound, many of the studies suffer from various limitations, which have been discussed in detail elsewhere.[31-33] Briefly, the limitations include lack of proper controls, population biases, short follow-up periods, small population sizes, inadequately controlled exposure conditions, and/or inadequate endpoints.

Because of the known susceptibility of the fetus to many environmental influences, current epidemiological research activity has been concentrated in the area of obstetrical ultrasound. Investigating for subtle and delayed effects of *in utero* exposure to ultrasound requires careful follow-up for a period of 5 to 8 years or possibly longer. A follow-up of children previously exposed *in utero*, a historical perspective study, could provide results in a shorter period of time at considerably less cost than exposing additional fetuses in the future and waiting several years before the data can be analyzed.

Table 1. Human studies of diagnostic ultrasound in pregnancy[1]

Principal investigator	Subjects	Controls	Mode	End point	Result
Kohorn (21)	20	same patients	p[2]	E.E.G.	no change
Bernstine (22)	720	none	p	prematurity	normal compared to U.S. Navy statistics
Hellman (23)	1114 normal	none	p & cw[3]	newborn exam	2.7% abnormality - "no effect"
Abdulla (24)	35	11	p & cw	chromosome exam (maternal and cord blood lymphocytes)	no increased aberrations
Serr (25)	10	10	cw	chromosome exam (fetal chromosomes obtained by amniocentesis)	some breaks but not statistically significant
Falus (26)	171	none	p	pediatric and anthropomorphic examination (1-3 years)	normal development
Falus (26)	10	10	p	chromosome exam (1-3 years)	no increased aberrations
Watts (27)	10	10	cw	chromosome exam (maternal & cord blood leukocytes)	no increased aberrations
Ikeuchi (28)	98	103	cw	chromosome exam (cultured fibroblasts of aborted fetuses)	no increased aberrations
David (29)	15	6	cw	fetal movement	increased movement
	15	same patients	cw	fetal movement	increased movement
Hertz (30)	13	same patients	cw	fetal movement	no increased movement

[1]Adapted from Ref. 32
[2]Pulsed ultrasound
[3]Continuous wave ultrasound

The Bureau of Radiological Health, under a contract with the University of Colorado Medical Center, has obtained epidemiological and statistical information on approximately 800 children, one half of whom were exposed to diagnostic ultrasound *in utero* during the period from 1968 to 1972. This information consists primarily of an exposure history of the mothers, birth records, and other clinical data concerning the fetuses. Follow-up information as to the physical, neurological, and clinical profile of the children between 6 and 11 years of age is also undergoing analysis.

An additional investigation is underway at the Health Sciences Center in Winnipeg, Canada.[33] In this study approximately 10,000 women who received ultrasound examination during pregnancy and 5,000 controls from the same time period are being identified and data collected from the hospital records. It is hoped to continue to observe these patients with examination for possible long-term effects.

The long-term goals of ultrasound epidemiological research are to ascertain the presence, or absence, of health effects due to human exposure to ultrasound and to determine, within reasonable and practicable limits, the degree of risk associated with such exposure. However, as in other problem areas (e.g., the effects of ionizing radiation), no single study can accomplish these goals. A program of collaborative research including well-designed and executed studies will be necessary to determine conclusively the extent of risk to human health posed by exposure to diagnostic ultrasound.

Laboratory Studies

Much of the early work in ultrasound bioeffects research has little direct applicability to possible adverse effects of diagnostic ultrasound. Early studies typically used average intensities that were quite high, relative to diagnostic ultrasound. Many of these studies examined endpoints that were representative of gross damage and were visually detectable. However, an examination of the available literature indicates that, in recent years, the level at which effects are being detected is decreasing. Also, many of the studies reporting effects at lower intensities involve subtle functional endpoints as opposed to gross pathological endpoints.

The following discussion of reported effects is not intended to be a comprehensive literature review but, rather, an examination of some of those studies reporting biological effects at spatial average, temporal average intensities of 500 mW/cm² or less, or studies that might indicate cumulative, synergistic, or additive effects of ultrasound exposure. Although at this time it has not been established which is the more important parameter of pulsed ultrasound, peak intensity or average intensity, all exposure intensities are reported as spatial and temporal average intensities.

Much of the current bioeffect information is controversial. Often the ultrasound dosimetry is inadequate, and most of the studies do not accurately mimic the conditions of the clinical situation. Other problems associated with the current data base include the lack of dose-effect data, the lack of threshold data, and the lack of data on long-term effects. In addition, much of the data is derived from exposure involving continuous wave ultrasound. The biological impact of short pulses of high intensity ultrasound, such as that used in pulse-echo ultrasound imaging, is little understood. These pulses may have a temporal peak intensity 1,000 times greater than the average intensity. Because of the many difficulties associated with the study of ultrasound bio-effects, evidence that is presented should be considered inconclusive in many cases until verified by other laboratories.

Structural and Physiological Effects

Many of the low intensity effects reported thus far are in the general area of structural and physiological effects (Table 2). Of these effects, the most sensitive endpoints appear to be functional as opposed to anatomical. Two of these low intensity reports involve the effect of diagnostic ultrasound units on the central nervous system. Increased levels of glutamic oxaloacetic trans-aminase (GOT) were found in the cerebrospinal fluid of dogs exposed to 1.5 mW/cm² pulsed ultrasound from a transducer placed over the intact scalp and skull for 9 hours.[34] Elevated concentrations of GOT are associated with cellular damage.[47] However, GOT analyses are subject to the influence of many stresses, and it is not clear that the control animals were restrained in the same manner as the exposed animals. It also has been reported that exposure to 3 mW/cm² pulsed ultrasound produced evoked potentials recorded by EEG electrodes implanted in the brains of anesthetized squirrel monkeys.[35] The evoked responses appeared immediately upon initiation of exposure and disappeared within 3 minutes but before the exposure ended.

In vitro cellular effects have also been associated with exposure to diagnostic ultrasound devices. A decreased incorporation of ³H-thymidine was observed in HeLa cells exposed to an intensity of 4 mW/cm², pulsed ultrasound, for 10 minutes.[36] Increased immunoreactivity to antinucleoside antibodies and apparent DNA repair synthesis in HeLa cells, and mor-phological transformation of mouse embryo cells have been reported after 20 minutes exposure to 17 mW/cm² pulsed ultrasound.[38] Other reported cellular effects of ultrasound exposure include altered viscoelastic proper-ties of Helodea cells after exposure to 40 mW/cm² for 3 minutes,[39] reduced growth of cultured human fibroblasts after a 1-hour exposure to 100 mW/cm²,[44] and a dose-related biphasic effect on ³H-thymidine uptake by human lymphocytes exposed in vitro with a standard Doppler fetal detector.[48]

A group in Great Britain has observed an increased rate of tissue regeneration, accompanied by an increased uptake of ^{3}H-thymidine, after sonicating experimentally produced surgical defects in rabbit ears with pulsed ultrasound. They found optimum growth stimulation after exposure to 100 mW/cm² administered in 5-minute treatments, 3 times a week.[43] Although there has been a reported reduction in the mitotic index of regenerating rat liver, as measured 30 hours after 5 minutes exposure to 60 mW/cm² and partial hepatectomy,[41] another group of investigators report no effect under similar exposure conditions.[49]

Table 2. Structural and physiological effects

Average[1] intensity (mW/cm²)	Total exposure time (min)	Test system	Effect observed
1.5 (p)[2]	360	canine CNS	increased GOT levels in cerebrospinal fluid (Ref. 34)
3 (p)	3[4]	primate	evoked EEG potentials (Ref. 35)
4 (p)	10	HeLa cells	decreased incorporation of nucleic acid precursor (Ref. 36)
8.9 (p)	5	mouse spleen	decreased immune response (Ref. 37)[6]
17 (p)	20	HeLa cells; mouse embryo cells	increased immunoreactivity, morphological transformation (Ref. 38)
40 (cw)[3]	3	Helodea cells	altered viscoelastic properties (Ref. 39)
50 (cw)	1.5[5]	rabbit eye	vascular changes (Ref. 40)
60 (cw)	5	rat liver	mitotic index (Ref. 41)[6]
65 (cw)	5	human blood	decreased in vitro clotting time (Ref. 42)
100 (cw)	5[5]	rabbit ear	enhanced wound healing (Ref. 43)
100 (p)	60	human fibroblasts	cell proliferation (Ref. 44)
500 (cw)	0.1	chick embryo	blood stasis (Ref. 45)
500 (cw)	2	canine bone marrow	hemorrhage (Ref. 46)

[1]Spatial and temporal average
[2]Pulsed ultrasound
[3]Continuous wave ultrasound
[4]Effect was transient; complete adaptation occurred with 3 minutes of exposure
[5]Multiple exposures
[6]Negative results reported at the same or greater average intensity (see text).

Several studies have reported that ultrasound can produce *in vitro* and *in vivo* hematological alterations. One of these studies demonstrated that platelet-rich plasma from human blood when exposed *in vitro* to 65 mW/cm² for 5 minutes exhibits a decreased recalcification time.[42] An earlier ophthalmological study reported vascular dilation at 50 mW/cm² exposure for 1.5 minutes.[40] Corneal erosions and erythrocytic extravasations were observed after repeated exposures to 50 mW/cm² for 1.5 minutes as well as after single exposures to 100 mW/cm² for 1 minute.[40] Another early study reported hemorrhaging in the bone marrow of canine femurs exposed to 500 mW/cm² for 2 minutes.[46] Blood stasis has been observed in the blood vessels of chick embryos exposed, under specialized conditions, to intensities as low as 500 mW/cm² for a few seconds.[45] The same investigators also observed damage to the endothelial lining of some blood vessels exposed under the same conditions, suggestive of lysosomal damage.[45]

There is little information on the possible effects of ultrasound on the immune system. One group of investigators reports an immunosuppressant effect in mice after exposure of the area of the spleen to 8.9 mW/cm² pulsed ultrasound for 5 minutes.[37] An attempt to repeat the study by another group of investigators did not confirm the finding.[50] However, because of the difficulties of detecting subtle immunological effects, the negative findings of one investigator do not necessarily invalidate the positive findings of another.

Developmental Effects

Because of the use of ultrasound to monitor and visualize the fetus, several researchers have attempted to investigate the effect of ultrasound on embryological development (Table 3). Preliminary results of work in progress indicate that neuromuscular development in rats, particularly coordinated functions, is delayed after *in utero* exposure to 10 mW/cm² for 5 minutes.[51] A group of behavioral scientists in Japan also reported delays in the maturation of neuromotor reflexes in rats, suggestive of changes in the functional development of the brain, after *in utero* exposure to 20 mW/cm² for 5 hours.[52] However, a recent study in the United States of the development of some of the same reflexes in mice exposed *in utero* to 50 or 500 mW/cm² of continuous wave ultrasound for 3 minutes indicated no significant differences between the exposed groups and the sham group.[58] A group of Japanese scientists has also reported findings that suggest that the emotional behavior of rats can be influenced by *in utero* exposure to 20 mW/cm² for 5 hours.[53] Another group of investigators in Japan found an increased in-

Table 3. Developmental effects

Average[1] intensity (mW/cm^2)		Total irradiation time (min)	Test system	Effect observed
10	(cw)[2]	5	rat	delayed neuromuscular development (Ref. 51)[3]
20	(cw)	300	rat	delayed neuromotor reflex development[3] (Ref. 52)
20	(cw)	300	rat	altered emotional behavior (Ref. 53)
40	(cw)	300	mouse	fetal abnormalities (Ref. 54)
125	(cw)	3	mouse	postpartum mortality[3] (Ref. 55)
75-750	(cw)	2	mouse	reduced fetal weight (Ref. 56)
500-5,000	(cw)	0.167-3	mouse	reduced fetal weight (Ref. 57)

[1]Spatial and temporal average
[2]Continuous wave ultrasound
[3]Negative results reported at the same or greater average intensity (see text).

cidence of congenital anomalies in mice after 5 hours of *in utero* exposure to a Doppler fetal heart monitor with a reported intensity of 40 mW/cm^2.[54] This study is somewhat controversial because of dosimetric uncertainties, the possibility that the effects could be the result of hyperthermia, and the fact that the anomaly incidence was significantly increased in one strain of mice and not in another.

There is a report of increased early postpartum mortality (up to the 21st day postpartum) of mouse pups exposed *in utero* on the 13th day of gestation to an intensity of 125 mW/cm^2 for 3 minutes.[55] Another group of investigators found no increased neonatal mortality, during the first 25 postpartum days, in mice exposed to 500 mW/cm^2 for up to 3 minutes.[59] There are several differences between these two studies; notably, the mice were exposed *in utero* at different stages of gestation. There have been reports of fetal weight reduction in mice exposed *in utero* to continuous wave ultrasound;[56,57] however, it is uncertain whether this is due to a direct effect on the fetus, or an effect on the dam (female parent) resulting from the exposure of a relatively large proportion of the animal under these experimental conditions.

Perhaps the greatest lack of information on low intensity ultrasound effects is in the area of genetics (Table 4). However, some of the lowest intensity effects reported to date do involve genetic material: decreased incorporation of a labeled nucleic acid precursor in HeLa cells exposed to 4 mW/cm² pulsed ultrasound,[36] and DNA repair synthesis in HeLa cells exposed to 17 mW/cm² pulsed ultrasound.[38] There have been reports of degradation of DNA in solution after exposure to 200 mW/cm² for 15 minutes[62] and 400 mW/cm² for 3 minutes.[63] A small but significant increase in the frequency of sister chromatid exchanges has been reported after exposure of human lymphocytes to approximately 5.0 mW/cm² pulsed ultrasound for 30 minutes.[60] Another laboratory reported no increase in the frequency of sister chromatid exchanges in human leukocytes after exposure to intensities as high as 36 W/cm².[64] However, the results of these studies are not directly comparable because of different experimental techniques and the fact that the former experiment employed pulsed ultrasound and the latter continuous wave ultrasound. The interpretation of sister chromatid exchanges and, particularly, the significance of this *in vitro* effect to the clinical situation are unclear.

Many investigators in the field of ultrasound suggest that these *in vitro* effects are the result of cavitation in the sonicated liquids. There is evidence that the dissolved gases in tissue can form bubbles under certain conditions (e.g., decompression sickness); the crucial question of whether or not bub-

Table 4. Genetic Effects

Average[1] intensity (mW/cm²)	Total irradiation time (min)	Test system	Effect observed
5 (p)[2]	30	human lymphocytes	sister chromatid exchange[4] (Ref. 60)
200 (cw)[3]	1	Vicia faba root	chromosomal aberrations (Ref. 61)
200 (cw)	15	calf thymus DNA	DNA strand degradation (Ref. 62)
400 (cw)	3	calf thymus & salmon sperm DNA	DNA strand degradation (Ref. 63)

[1]Spatial and temporal average
[2]Pulsed ultrasound
[3]Continuous wave ultrasound
[4]Negative results also reported at the same or greater average intensity (see text).

bles of resonant size can form in tissue under clinical diagnostic conditions of ultrasound exposure has yet to be answered.

Although there have been no verified reports of "classical" chromosome aberrations due to diagnostic or therapeutic levels of ultrasound, chromosome anomalies of another type have been observed. A Czechoslovakian investigator reported chromosome and chromatid abnormalities in bean (*Vicia faba*) roots after exposure to 200 mW/cm² for 1 minute.[61] A group at the University of Rochester, New York, who reported chromosome damage in bean (*Vicia faba*) roots after exposure to somewhat greater intensities,[65,66] suggest that other researchers may not have observed these particular types of aberrations because of scoring technique. The "standard" technique for scoring metaphases for chromosome aberrations selects against mitotic figures that are not well spread; thus bridged and agglomerated mitotic figures may be ignored. However, again, the significance of these effects to the clinical situation is unclear; it is the opinion of some investigators that plant cells possess structural characteristics that enhance the occurrence of cavitation.

Studies on hereditable genetic alterations induced by ultrasound have yielded negative reports to date, including a study in mice by a well-recognized radiation geneticist.[67] However, few mammalian systems have been tested, and the mouse study [67] shows considerable variability of the data in some of the tests performed and was conducted with rather small sample sizes.[68]

Other Effects

The question of whether or not ultrasound-induced effects accumulate is of vital importance when assessing the safety of ultrasound. Most of the work in this area has been concerned with the summation of short pulses of ultrasound as opposed to the accumulation of exposures. Early investigators, using the frog spinal cord, showed that accumulation of effects from repeated pulses was possible with a 50% duty factor.[69] Another group of investigators exposed the rat spinal cord to various regimens of pulsed ultrasound and found that a constant accumulated exposure time would produce vascular damage when the duty factor was as small as 2.5%.[70] One of the few reports of the effect of fractionated exposures has revealed that splitting the exposure into two fractions, separated by 24 hours, did not alter the observed effect, a reduction in growth rate of irradiated bean (*Vicia faba*) roots.[71]

Although there have been conflicting reports concerning the synergistic or additive effects of ultrasound and x rays for destroying tumors,[72,73] there have been unrefuted reports that ultrasound and x rays reduced the electrophoretic mobility of tumor cells in an additive manner [74] and that ultrasound can enhance the x-ray induced inactivation of cultured hamster cells.[75] It also has been reported that hypoxia and ultrasound exhibit synergism by decreasing the exposure time required to produce hemorrhage in the rat spinal cord.[70]

Summary

In summary, there are many deficiencies and gaps in the current data base for ultrasound-induced bioeffects. More information is needed on the effects of low intensity ultrasound, the effects of pulsed ultrasound, the relationship between peak intensities and average intensities of pulsed ultrasound, the possibility of cumulative effects, and the possibility of long-term effects. Also, very little of the data, either positive or negative, has been verified by other laboratories. Although there is presently no evidence to indicate that diagnostic ultrasound involves a significant risk, the evidence is insufficient to justify an unqualified acceptance of safety. The potential for acute adverse effects has not been systematically explored, and the potential for delayed effects has been virtually ignored.

Because of the difficulties involved in searching for and defining potential risks from exposure to low levels of chemicals, radiation, or other forms of energy, it is unreasonable to expect that in the near future, the degree of risk, if any, will be clearly defined for diagnostic ultrasound. As in other areas (e.g., the effects of ionizing radiation) no single study, epidemiological or experimental, can accomplish this goal. In the meantime, a prudent public health policy calls for judicious use of diagnostic ultrasound, using it only when diagnostic benefits to patients are indicated, and keeping any exposure to diagnostic ultrasound as low as practicable, consistent with its intended purpose.

REFERENCES

1. Nyborg W L. *Physical mechanisms for biological effects of ultrasound.* HEW Publication (FDA) no. 78–8062, Sept. 1977.

2. Fry F J. *Ultrasound: Its applications in medicine and biology.* New York, Elsevier Publishing Co, 1978.

3. Goss S A, Johnston R L, Dunn F. Comprehensive compilation of empirical ultrasonic properties of mammalian tissues. *J Acoust Soc Am* 64:423-457, 1978.

4. Chivers R C, Parry R J. Ultrasonic velocity and attenuation in mammalian tissues. *J Acoust Soc Am* 63:940-953, 1978.

5. Muir T G, Carstensen E L. Prediction of nonlinear acoustic effects of biomedical frequencies and intensities. *Ultrasound Med Biol* 6:341-355, 1980.

6. Muir T G. Nonlinear effects in acoustic imaging. In *Proceedings of the 9th International Symposium on Acoustical Imaging*. Wang K (ed). New York, Plenum Press, 1980.

7. Flynn H G. Physics of acoustic cavitation in liquids. In *Physical acoustics*. Mason W P (ed). New York, Academic Press, 1964, vol. 1B.

8. Apfel R E. The tensile strength of liquids. *Sci Am* 227 (6):58–71, 1972.

9. Eller A, Flynn H G. Rectified diffusion during nonlinear pulsations of cavitation bubbles. *J Acoust Soc Am* 37:493–503, 1965.

10. Carstensen E L, Child S Z, Law W K, et al. Cavitation as a mechanism for the biological effects of ultrasound on plant roots. *J Acoust Soc Am* 66:1285–1291, 1979.

11. Child, S Z, Carstensen E L, Lam S K. Effects of ultrasound on *Drosophila*: III. Exposure of larvae to low-temporal-average-intensity, pulsed irradiation. *Ultrasound Med Biol* 7:167–173, 1981.

12. Harvey E N, Barnes D K, McElroy W D, et al. Bubble formation in animals. I. Physical factors. *J Cell Comp Physiol* 24:1–23, 1944.

13. ter Haar G R, Daniels S. Evidence for ultrasonically induced cavitation *in vivo*. *Phys Med Biol* 26:1145–1149, 1981.

14. Nyborg W L, Miller D L, Gershoy A. Physical consequences of ultrasound in plant tissues and other bio-systems. In *Fundamental and applied aspects of nonionizing radiation*. Michaelson S M, Miller M W (eds). New York, Plenum Press, 1975.

15. Williams A R, Hughes D E, Nyborg W L. Hemolysis near a transversely oscillating wire. *Science* 169:871–873, 1970.

16. ter Haar G, Wyard S J. Blood cell banding in ultrasonic standing wave field: A physical analysis. *Ultrasound Med Biol* 4:111–123, 1978.

17. O'Brien W D. In *Ultrasound: Its applications in medicine and biology*. Vol 3, Part 1. Fry F J (ed). New York, Elsevier Publishing Co., 1978.

18. American Institute of Ultrasound in Medicine (AIUM) Standards Committee. *Recommended nomenclature*, Physics and Engineering, Oklahoma City, AIUM Executive Office, 1980.

19. Stewart H S. Diagnostic ultrasonic output levels and quality assurance measurement techniques. In *Proceedings of the 11th Annual National Conference in Radiation Control*. HHS Publication no. (FDA) 81–8054, 1981.

20. Christman C L. Average dose absorbed by biological specimens in a diffuse ultrasonic exposure field. *J Acoust Soc Am* 70:946–954, 1981.

21. Kohorn E L, Pritchard H, Hobbins J. The safety of clinical ultrasonic examination. *Obstet Gynecol* 29:272–274, 1962.

22. Bernstine R L. Safety studies with ultrasonic Doppler technique, a clinical follow-up of patients and tissue culture study. *Obstet Gynecol* 34:707, 1969.

23. Hellman L, Duffus G, Donald I. Safety of diagnostic ultrasound in obstetrics. *Lancet* p 1133–1135, May 30, 1970.

24. Abdulla U, Dewhurst C, Campbell S, et al. Effect of diagnostic ultrasound on maternal and fetal chromosomes. *Lancet* p 7729, Oct. 16, 1971.

25. Serr D M, Padeh B, Zakett H, et al. Studies on the effects of ultrasonic waves on the fetus. In *Proceedings of the 2nd European Congress in Perinatal Medicine*. Huntingford P J, Beard R W, Hytten, et al (eds). London, 1971.

26. Falus M, Korany G, Sobel M, et al. Follow-up studies on infants examined by ultrasound during the fetal age. *Orrosi Hetilap* ll3:2119–2121, 1972. (Translated from the Hungarian.)

27. Watts P, Stewart C. The effect of fetal heart monitoring by ultrasound on maternal and fetal chromosomes. *J Obstet Gynaecol Br Commonw* 79:715–716, 1972.

28. Ikeuchi T, Sasaki M, Oshimuoa M, et al. Ultrasound and embryonic chromosomes. *Br Med J* p 112, Jan. 13, 1973.

29. David H, Weaver J B, Pearson J F. Doppler ultrasound and fetal activity. *Br Med J* 2:62–64, 1975.

30. Hertz R H, Timor-Tritsch I, Dierker L J, et al. Continuous ultrasound and fetal movement. *Am J Obstet Gynecol* 135:152–154, 1979.

31. Landau E. Are there ultrasonic dangers for the unborn? *J Invest Radiol* 1:27–31, 1973.

32. Scheidt P C. *Human studies of diagnostic ultrasound in pregnancy.* Bureau of Radiological Health Presentation at the Panel on Review of Obstetrical-Gynecological Devices. Washington, DC, Feb. 3, 1975.

33. Scheidt P C, Lundin F E. Investigations for effects of intrauterine ultrasound on humans. In *Proceedings of a Symposium on Biological Effects and Characterizations of Ultrasound Sources.* Hazzard D G, Litz M L (eds). HEW Publication no. (FDA) 78-8048, 1977.

34. Tsutsumi Y, Sano K, Kuwabara T, et al. A new portable echo-encephalograph, using ultrasonic transducers; and its clinical application. *Med Electron Biol Eng* 2:21–29, 1964.

35. Hu J H, Ulrich W D. Effects of low-intensity ultrasound on the central nervous system of primates. *Aviat Space Environ Med* 47:640–643, 1976.

36. Prasad N. Ultrasound and mammalian DNA. *Lancet* p 1181, May 29, 1976.

37. Anderson D W, Barrett J T. Ultrasound: A new immunosuppressant. *Clin Immunol Immunopathol* 14:18–29, 1979.

38. Liebeskind D, Bases R, Elequin F, et al. Diagnostic ultrasound: Effects on DNA and growth patterns of animal cells. *Radiology* 131:177–184, 1979.

39. Johnsson A, Lindvall A. Effects of low-intensity ultrasound on viscous properties of Helodea cells. *Naturwissenschaften* 56:40, 1969.

40. Jankowiak J, Majewska H, Majewski H. Ophthalmologic and histologic changes in rabbit eyes induced by ultrasound *Am J Phys Med* 44:70–77, 1965.

41. Kremkau F W, Witcofski R L. Mitotic reduction in rat liver exposed to ultrasound. *J Clin Ultrasound* 2:123–126, 1974.

42. Williams A R, O'Brien W D, Coller B S. Exposure to ultrasound decreases the recalcification time of platelet rich plasma. *Ultrasound Med Biol* 2:113–118, 1976.

43. Dyson M, Pond J, Joseph J, et al. Stimulation of tissue regeneration by pulsed plane-wave ultrasound. *IEEE Trans Sonics Ultrasonics* SU-17:133–140, 1970.

44. Loch E G, Fischer A, Kuwert E. Effect of diagnostic and therapeutic intensities of ultrasonics on normal and malignant human cells *in vitro. Am J Obstet Gynecol* 110:456–460, 1971.

45. Dyson M, Pond J. Effects of ultrasound on circulation. *Physiotherapy* 59:284–287, 1973.

46. Bender L F, Janes J M, Herrick J F. Histological studies following exposure of bone to ultrasound. *Arch Phys Med Rehab* 35:555–559, 1954.

47. Frankel S, Reitman S, Sonnenwirth A C (eds). *Gradwohl's clinical laboratory methods and diagnosis* (7th ed) Vol 2, p 1973, St Louis, C V Mosby Co, 1970.

48. Fung H, Cheung K, Lyons E A, et al. The effect of low dose ultrasound on human peripheral lymphocyte function *in vitro.* In *Ultrasound in medicine.* Vol 4. White D, Lyons E A (eds). New York, Plenum Press, 1976.

49. Miller M W, Kaufman G E, Cataldo F L, et al. Absence of mitotic reduction in regenerating rat livers exposed to ultrasound. *J Clin Ultrasound* 4:169–172, 1976.

50. Child S Z, Hare J D, Carstensen E L, et al. Test for effects of diagnostic levels of ultrasound on the immune response of mice. *Clin Immunol Immunopathol* 18:299–302, 1981.

51. Sikov M R, Hildebrand B P, Stearns J D. Postnatal sequelae of ultrasound exposure at fifteen days in gestation in the rat (work in progress). Third World Congress of Ultrasonics in Medicine, Aug 3–7, 1976.

52. Murai N, Hoshi K, Nakamura T. Effects of diagnostic ultrasound irradiated during fetal stage on development of orienting behavior and reflex ontogeny in rats. *Tohoku J Exp Med* 116:17–24, 1975.

53. Murai N, Hoshi K, Kang C, et al. Effects of diagnostic ultrasound irradiated during foetal stage on emotional and cognitive behavior in rats, *Tohoku J Exp Med* 117:225–235, 1975.

54. Shoji R E, Shimizu T, Matsuda S. An experimental study on the effect of low intensity ultrasound on developing mouse embryos. *Teratology* 6:119, 1976.

55. Curto K A. Early post-partum mortality following ultrasonic radiation. In *Ultrasound in medicine.* Vol 2. White D, Barnes R (eds). New York, Plenum Press, 1976.

56. Stratmeyer M E, Pinkavitch F Z, Simmons L R, et al. *In utero* effects of ultrasound exposure in mice. *Proceedings of the 26th Annual Meeting of the American Institute of Ultrasound in Medicine*, p 121, 1981.

57. O'Brien W D Jr. Ultrasonically induced fetal weight reduction in mice. In *Ultrasound in medicine*. Vol 2. White D, Barnes R (eds). New York, Plenum Press, 1976.

58. Brown NT, Galloway WD, Henton WW. Reflex development following *in utero* exposure to ultrasound. In *Proceedings of the 26th Annual Meeting of the American Institute of Ultrasound in Medicine*, p 119, 1981.

59. Edmonds PD, Stolzenberg SJ, Torbit CA, et al. Post partum survival of mice exposed *in utero* to ultrasound. *J Acoust Soc Am* 66:590–593, 1979.

60. Liebeskind D, Bases B, Mendez F, et al. Sister chromatid exchanges in human lymphocytes after exposure to diagnostic ultrasound. *Science* 205:1273–1275, 1979.

61. Slotova J, Karpfel Z, Hrazdira H. Chromosome aberrations caused by the effect of ultrasound in the meristematic cells of *Vicia faba*. *Biol Plantarum* 9:49–55, 1967.

62. Galperin-Lamaitre H, Kirsch-Volders M, Levi S. Fragmentation of purified mammalian DNA molecules by ultrasound below human therapeutic doses, *Humangenetik* 29:61–66, 1975.

63. Hill CR, Clark PR, Growe MR, et al. Biophysical effects of cavitation in a 1 MHz ultrasonic beam, Ultrasonics for Industry Conference Papers 1969, pp 26–30, 1969.

64. Morris SM, Palmer CG, Fry FJ, et al. Effect of ultrasound on human leucocytes: Sister chromatid exchange analysis. *Ultrasound Med Biol* 4:253–258, 1978.

65. Cataldo FL, Miller MW, Gregory WD, et al. A description of ultrasonically-induced chromosomal anomalies in *Vicia faba*. *Radiation Bot* 13:211–213, 1973.

66. Gregory WD, Miller MW, Carstensen EL, et al. Nonthermal effects of 2 MHz ultrasound on the growth cytology of *Vicia faba* roots. *Br J Radiol* 47:122–129, 1974.

67. Lyon MF, Simpson GM. An investigation into the possible genetic hazards of ultrasound. *Br J Radiol* 47:712–722, 1974.

68. Stratmeyer ME. Genetic effects of ultrasound. Presented at the Ad Hoc Meeting on Ultrasound Bioeffects and Measurements, Rockville, MD, Apr 9 10, 1976.

69. Fry WJ, Wulff VJ, Tucker D, et al. Physical factors involved in ultrasonically induced changes in living systems. I. Identification of nontemperature effects. *J Acoust Soc Am* 22:867–876, 1950.

70. Taylor KJW, Pond JB. A study of the production of haemorrhagic injury and paraplegia in rat spinal cord by pulsed ultrasound of low megahertz frequencies in the context of the safety for clinical usage. *Br J Radiol* 45:343–353, 1972.

71. Bleaney BI, Oliver R. The effect of irradiation of *Vicia faba*, *Radiation Bot* 13:211–213, 1973.

72. Woeber K. The effect of ultrasound in the treatment of cancer. In *Ultrasonic energy*, Kelley E (ed). Urbana, IL, University of Illinois Press, 1965.

73. Clarke PR, Hill CR, Adams K. Synergism between ultrasound and x rays in tumour therapy. *Br J Radiol* 43:97–99, 1970.

74. Repacholi MH, Woodcock JP, Newman DL, et al. Interaction of low intensity ultrasound and ionizing radiation with tumour cell surface. *Phys Med Biol* 16:221–227, 1971.

75. Todd P, Schroy CB. X ray inactivation of cultured mammalian cells: Enhancement by ultrasound. *Radiology* 113:445–447, 1974.

RECEIVED: APRIL, 1982
REVISED & ACCEPTED: AUGUST, 1982

EXTERNAL CEPHALIC VERSION

Brigitte Jordan

Breech presentation, which occurs in 3% to 4% of all deliveries, presents a problem for obstetrical management, since it is associated with substantially higher fetal and maternal risk than delivery from a vertex presentation. In contemporary American obstetrics two standard management strategies are accepted: breech delivery for selected patients and, increasingly, cesarean section. This chapter is concerned with a third alternative: external cephalic version (ECV), the manipulative transabdominal conversion of the breech to a cephalic presentation.

Both of the currently standard management strategies have their drawbacks. Vaginal breech delivery is associated with a high perinatal mortality, which reaches three to four times the rate of vertex presentations, even when the greater incidence of prematurity and congenital abnormalities is controlled for.[8,26,32] Surviving infants show lower Apgar scores and a greater incidence of birth injuries, mental retardation, cerebral palsy, and learning disabilities, although it is not clear what proportion of this morbidity is due to prematurity and what proportion is contributed by the route of delivery. Nevertheless, the hazards contingent on route of delivery suggest that perinatal outcome would be improved if vaginal breech delivery could be avoided.

Considerations of this sort constitute one reason why surgical delivery is rapidly becoming the preferred solution for the problem of breech presentation. Today, breech presentation constitutes one of the three most frequent indications for cesarean section in the United States. Many institutions report delivering 60% to 90% of their breech presentations in this way.[22] Especially for younger practitioners, many of whom are increasingly unskilled in the art of breech delivery, the figure is closer to 100%. If one considers that breech as an indication for primary section also contributes to the number of repeat cesareans, it becomes abundantly clear that this type of fetal presentation constitutes a significant factor in the substantial and continuing rise of the cesarean section rate in the United States.

Although cesarean section clearly lowers perinatal mortality when compared with vaginal breech delivery,[4,14,25] it still carries a higher risk for the baby when compared with the vaginal delivery of a cephalic presentation.

Moreover, cesarean section is associated with increased maternal mortality which, although low, nevertheless ranges from two to thirty times that found among vaginally delivered mothers,[1,22] a fetal mortality almost triple that of nonsurgical deliveries even when gestational age is controlled for,[22] increased incidence of respiratory problems of the newborn, high incidence of maternal infection, pain and complications associated with major surgery, lengthy postsurgical disability, maternal psychological disturbances and interruption of mother-infant and father-infant attachment.[39]

Delivery from breech, whether vaginal or abdominal, is thus always associated with higher risk for mother and child than the birth of a vertex-presenting baby. External cephalic version (ECV), by substituting the vertex for the breech, promises to transform some substantial proportion of the high-risk breech population into a low-risk cephalic population. This chapter is devoted to a critical examination of this promise.

The data on which the present discussion is based are derived from a review of the American and European medical literature, on personal observation of ECVs during crosscultural research on perinatal practices, and on discussions with experienced lay and medical practitioners as well as with women who have undergone versions. It should be noted that whereas most of what follows applies equally to other types of malpresentations, particularly transverse lie, my concern here, unless otherwise noted, will be specifically with singleton breech fetuses.

Some Historical and Crosscultural Considerations

During the first decades of the 20th century, ECV was widely practiced in the United States as well as in Europe and elsewhere, with a general agreement that version was considerably less dangerous than breech delivery. By the 1950s, however, the practice had fallen into disuse in the United States and presently is rarely practiced, much less taught in medical schools or obstetrical residencies.

Although ECV has almost died out in the United States, it is alive and well in other parts of the world. The largest number of versions is probably performed by traditional birth attendants in developing countries. But it is also commonly practiced by midwives with varying levels of training the world over and, maybe most relevantly for American practice, is frequent in the technologically sophisticated obstetrics of Europe, in countries such as Holland, Sweden, and Germany. These countries are industrialized, enjoy a high standard of living, and share with the United States a scientific foundation for their obstetrics. Practitioners in such countries, in contrast with the poorer regions of the world, also have access to the range of resources provided by modern medical technology, pharmacology, and surgery, so that it cannot be argued that their high regard for ECV is due to lack of facilities and technical expertise.

It is interesting to observe that in obstetrical communities where ECV is accepted and routinely practiced—and that was as true for the earlier American period as it is in present-day Europe—advocates of ECV maintain that it is associated with little risk and should constitute the conservative method of first choice. They argue that version is, logically and in their experience, superior to either breech delivery or cesarean section. In countries where is it not accepted, on the other hand, practitioners believe with equal conviction that the risks associated with ECV are too high and justify abandoning it in favor of, nowadays, surgical delivery. As we will see, no compelling argument can be constructed by either side on the basis of evidence reported in the biomedical literature. In the last analysis, the use or condemnation of ECV may have more to do with cultural notions about the nature of pregnancy and birth than with "objective" evidence of benefits and risks.

If we look at the practice of ECV worldwide, it becomes apparent that there are three major approaches to version. The first, historically as well as in frequency, is what I will call "the traditional approach." This is version without technological aids of any kind, performance of which relies exclusively on the manipulative skills of the attendant. The second type I will call "the conventional medical approach." It requires only minimal technology, such as a stethoscope for monitoring the fetal heart. This is the method which was used by American practitioners until version was supplanted by the current management options. It is also the method used by trained European midwives and by the majority of physicians who do versions. The third approach, "tocolytic version," is a very recent development, first proposed by German physicians in 1975. Its major feature is the use of tocolytic (uterine-relaxant) drugs, which allow the performance of ECV very close to term. Tocolytic ECV, in contrast with the traditional and the conventional approaches, requires sophisticated obstetrical technology and the ability to perform immediate cesarean section.

Nature and Quality of the Data Regarding ECV

The central question in regard to ECV is, simply: What are the risks of the procedure? Are they negligible, as is argued by its advocates, or does the external manipulation of the fetus add such substantial risk to a pregnancy that the final outcome is no better, or possibly even worse, than if the baby had been delivered from breech. Unfortunately, neither the advocates nor the critics of ECV can point to much in the way of scientifically respectable evidence for their position, and this is true for practitioners of the conventional medical approach as well as for those utilizing the more recent tocolytic method. (For versions performed by traditional birth attendants in third world countries, no systematically collected data exist at all.)

Every one of the studies that will be cited in this chapter is open to multiple criticism on methodological grounds. The most glaring deficiency is inadequate research design. With a single exception,[38] none of the investigators has employed the standard research design for the production of scientific evidence: prospective studies with randomized clinical trials. In addition, many of the studies, in particular those of the tocolytic approach, are based on inordinately small samples. This is a grave problem, since the expected rate of occurrence for any one complication is small, and to show statistical significance for small increases in risk, large samples are required. Furthermore, practitioners do not agree on which risk variables are important, nor on how to operationalize those which they do investigate. It is, for example, by no means clear what evidence should count as placental damage, or cord complications, or even what constitutes a successful version.

It is thus probably fair to say that whereas the medical literature contains a large number of reports on ECV, the quality of the data presented is highly suspect. The net effect of the deficiencies just outlined (and others not even mentioned, such as questions of reliability and validity), is that extreme caution must be exercised when interpreting outcome statistics. It is important to keep in mind that methodologically unassailable studies of ECV have not been done and that a scientific assessment of the risks and benefits of version still awaits large-sample research that is designed and executed according to the canons of scientific investigation.

Effectiveness of ECV in Reducing Breech Incidence, Prematurity, and Section Rate

One of the few issues around ECV for which there are reasonably convincing data concerns the question of whether version is effective in lowering the incidence of breech presentation at the time of delivery. It is sometimes argued that the fetuses which can be turned by external manipulation are precisely those which, with time, would have turned spontaneously, so that nothing is gained by the version. This is clearly a consequential issue. If it is the case that version is ineffectual, then mother/fetus pairs on whom version is attempted are merely subjected to additional risk, no matter how small. If, on the other hand, ECV does lower the incidence of breech presentation, some number of infants will escape the hazards of breech delivery or cesarean section. As will be shown later, there can be no reasonable doubt that a consistent policy of version reduces the number of infants delivered from breech, either vaginally or abdominally.

It has also been argued, with less supporting data, that version will reduce the incidence of prematurity. It is well known that prematurity and breech presentation are associated, but the causal direction of the relationship is by no means clear. It may be possible that prematurely occurring labor simply catches more fetuses which have not yet had time to turn by themselves. On the other hand, it may also be the case that breech presentation itself causes premature labor because of increased stimulation of the lower uterine segment by the fetal legs and mobile breech. Ranney[31] suggests that ECV may actually protect against premature labor by substituting the rounder, less irritating vertex. In his series, the prematurity rate of babies delivered from breech or transverse presentation was 17.77%, whereas those delivered vertex after version had a prematurity rate of 2.97%. Others[15,33,37] also consider it possible that version, far from causing premature labor, actually reduces its incidence.

In spite of the fact that prematurity reduction remains an open question, the reduction of breech presentation per se is not, as is conceded even by opponents of ECV.[3] The following figures should be read against a normal breech incidence of 3% to more than 4% at the time of delivery.

The greatest reduction in breech incidence was achieved by Ranney,[31] a persistent and skillful practitioner of ''the gentle art of cephalic version.'' Of 860 singleton breech or transverse fetuses who were under his care prenatally (allowing for early and if necessary multiple attempts at version), he was able to convert 806 to vertex, reducing thereby the incidence of malpresentation to 0.56% among his 4,817 obstetrical patients. Hibbard and Schumann[15] report data from a ''natural laboratory,'' a close-knit group of physicians who dealt with the same patient population and followed the same management strategies, except that one of them systematically attempted ECV on all breech presentations. They note a breech incidence of 2% in 4,043 singleton pregnancies cared for by the physician who did versions, compared with 3.5% in the patients delivered by the other physicians during the same time at the same hospital. In a Finnish obstetrical population, breech incidence at birth was 4.5% of 15,279 singleton pregnancies immediately prior to the study period and 2.9% of 18,783 singletons during the period when ECV was consistently attempted.[40] Using the tocolytic approach, Saling and Muller-Holve[34] report a reduction to 1.6% from 3.8% for singletons weighing more than 2,500 grams, and a Swedish study shows a reduction from 2.8% to 1.6% for singletons excluding stillbirths.[7]

Looking at these and other authors' figures, it appears that a reasonably consistently applied policy of version, even with varying inclusion criteria, will lead to a reduction of breech incidence at birth by something between 40% and 60% or more.

The implications of this fact for lowering the section rate will depend on local management strategies for breech, but can be expected to be particularly substantial where malpresentations are routinely delivered by cesarean. In a German institution, where the policy is cesarean section for all breeches, 15 of 23 patients on whom version was attempted were spared surgery.[18] Swedish investigators, who designed a study specifically to examine the possibility of section reduction in an institution with an average cesarean rate of 50%, argue that they saved 18 of their 37 successful version patients from abdominal delivery, since only one of them required a cesarean. In the United States, Van Dorsten and co-workers, in the randomized prospective study mentioned earlier, found that the cesarean rate was 74% in the control group of 23 women who underwent standard breech management, 75% in their failure group of 8 women, and occurred in only 1 case (6%) among the 17 women on whom version had been performed successfully.[38] A number of other authors report large differences in the cesarean rate between successes and failures, but they neglect to give information on how these rates compare with the obstetrical population at large or with standardly managed breeches.[2,19,31,40] Since ECV is clearly effective in reducing breech incidence at term and since breech is a major indication for cesarean section, it will always lower the frequency of abdominal delivery in any population in which ECV is consistently performed.

The Timing of ECV and the Issue of Success Rates

It is common knowledge that many fetuses present as breech some time during pregnancy and that most of these turn spontaneously before they reach term. Thus the number of breeches encountered in any obstetrical population decreases steadily (although not uniformly) from about 25% around the 20th week, to between 3% and 4% at term. It follows that if version is done early, the success rate is going to be high because the pool of fetuses on whom version is attempted contains a large proportion who would have turned by themselves. If version is done late, on the other hand, the success rate is computed on a pool from which most spontaneous versions have already been removed, so that the proportion of failures will be increased.

Two philosophies exist concerning the optimal timing of ECV that generate different success rates. The first advocates early version, since the procedure is clearly easier to perform with less advanced gestation. At that time there is plenty of amniotic fluid, the uterus is not tonic or irritable, the mother feels only slight discomfort, and anesthesia or tocolysis is not likely to be necessary. Traditional birth attendants and practitioners of the conservative medical persuasion tend to advocate early version, some of them as early as the 6th month,[13,15,23,33] and definitely by the 28th week.[20,29,31,35] These practitioners are fully aware that many of their successes will revert to breech and that up to one third of the procedures will have to be repeated. Early and persistent attempts continued up to and including labor make sense where ECV is considered a low-risk procedure. The success rate with this approach may go as high as 97%,[23,31] and is generally well above 80%.

In contrast to the "start early and keep at it" philosophy of traditional and conventional practitioners, advocates of tocolytic ECV place the procedure very close to term to avoid doing it unnecessarily. This line of thinking makes sense if it is assumed that ECV carries more than negligible risk. Success rates for late version dates, that is after the 37th week, are more in the vicinity of 70%.[7,18,34,38]

Although the literature exhibits a pervasive preoccupation with success rates, such figures are close to meaningless without controlling for gestational age, and their prevalence in the literature probably has more to do with the ease of collecting them than with any comparative utility. Such figures cannot be used for arguing for the relative efficacy of one ECV method versus another. In particular, the argument that early ECV is better than late *because of the higher success rate* is fallacious (although one might want to make that argument on other grounds). More appropriate data for assessing success are the effects of ECV on the obstetrical population at term, that is, the data on effectiveness of ECV in reducing breech incidence, which were discussed earlier.

Potential Risks of ECV

There are many studies noting no fetal mortality attributable to ECV.[5,7,13,18,19,27,31,33-35] Others report some deaths whose attribution to version is questionable,[15,20,29] but even where fetal mortality occurs, it is in every case a fraction of what would be expected in breech delivery.[6,12,35,37] The only equivocal results are reported by Bradley-Watson,[3] who found a 0.9% fetal mortality attributable to version. He argues that in modern, well-equipped institutions with a liberal cesarean section policy, where only favorable cases come to breech delivery, the perinatal loss is rarely as high as 1%. He concludes that a policy of routine version has decreasing value today.

Of the potential risks of ECV, the most serious are placental trauma and cord compromise. Evidence for damage to the placenta may consist of anything from slight and transient spotting, indicating partial and often inconsequential premature separation, to complete abruptio placentae with disastrous results.

The majority of investigators note either no vaginal bleeding at all or transient light spotting with no effect on mother or child.[5,6,12,13,15,23,29,31,33–36,38] Ranney[31] finds no difference in the rate of premature separation of the placenta between his version patients and his entire obstetrical population. Negative results are rare, but there is one study which shows a fairly high incidence of antepartum hemorrhage (3%),[3] and among tocolytic practitioners several cesarean sections were necessary because of premature separation.[18,19]

A persistent argument in the ECV literature concerns the possibility that the procedure loops the cord around the baby's neck, leading to fetal distress either at the time of version or as the head descends during labor. Fetal distress during version is easily controlled by checking the fetal heart before and after the procedure and by returning the fetus to its previous position if abnormalities are noted.[15,28,29,33] It appears that the fetal heart is almost always a bit slow after version, but recovery occurs quickly and regularly and reversals are rarely necessary. With the tocolytic approach, version is performed close to term, and immediate cesarean section is an option in case of serious fetal distress.[19] There is no good evidence that version causes a higher incidence of nuchal cord than normal. After all, if ECV is likely to wrap a cord around the neck, it is just as likely to unwrap a preexisting loop. At any rate, successful version eliminates the substantially higher rate of cord complications associated with breech delivery, where cord prolapse is between three and twenty times (depending on type of breech) as frequent as in cephalic presentation.

In addition to placental trauma and cord compromise, there are sporadic reports of premature labor, premature rupturing of membranes, and compound presentations resulting from ECV.[18,34] Because the frequencies are so low, comparison of these rare complications with their incidence in a nontreated population is not feasible. In regard to premature labor, one might keep in mind that this condition is associated with breech presentation per se, so that it may be impossible to say whether performing a version was itself causative or merely precipitated an early labor that would have occurred anyway.

A recent concern that does not appear in the earlier literature is the possibility of fetomaternal transfusion. This carries the risk of hemolytic disease of the newborn consequent to iso-immunization of an Rh-negative mother with an Rh-positive fetus. Gentle version seems to carry no increased risk in this regard,[31,38] but as the force of manipulation is increased, fetomaternal hemorrhage is more likely to occur.[21] The most negative results are reported by Lehmann and co-workers,[19] who found fetal blood cells in 9 of 28 patients (32%). Four of these had macrotransfusions of between 30 and 50 ml, and in each of these cases an abnormal fetal electrocardiogram was evident after version. These massive hemorrhages may well be related to the version method employed, which included tocolysis, cesarean section readiness, and in the majority of cases, anesthesia.

Beyond the independent contributions of anesthesia and tocolysis, it appears that the underlying factor in many of these complications is the duration and force of manipulation. The incidence and severity of placental trauma and fetomaternal hemorrhage appear to rise with advanced gestational age, when version fails, with the use of anesthesia, if the placenta is implanted on the anterior wall of the uterus (which restricts the maneuverable field), if labor has begun, and under all conditions which lead to applying undue force.

The Traditional Approach to ECV

Apart from sporadic mention,[17] there is little in the anthropological (not to speak of the biomedical) literature about ECV in traditional societies. It appears, however, that version is common wherever traditional ethno-obstetrical systems have a strong empirical orientation. In the course of crosscultural research on childbirth and perinatal practices,[10,16] my collaborators and I have had numerous occasions to observe ECVs as they were performed by a Maya Indian midwife in Yucatan, Mexico. Our impression is that the way Maya Indians do versions is fairly typical of the methods of other traditional birth attendants. We made videotapes of four versions performed by the midwife who is our prime informant, one of which is available in edited form.[9]

"Turning the baby" is a routine practice in the region and constitutes an important element in the collection of traditional midwifery arts and practices. In government-sponsored training courses for traditional birth attendants, version is condemned as too dangerous and it is suggested that mid-wives bring women with breech presentation to the nearest hospital for possible surgical delivery.

In Yucatan, the midwife is a woman of the community who shares with her clients common notions about how the body functions, what constitutes a "normal" pregnancy, what constitutes "trouble" in pregnancy and birth, and what to do if trouble indeed arises. She performs versions in the course of a special massage, which she routinely administers during her regular prenatal visits.

The woman lies on a blanket on the dirt floor of her hut, with the mid-wife seated on a low stool to one side of her (Fig. 1). During the first few movements of the massage, the midwife ascertains the position of the fetus. She will try to move it with the head leading, maintaining it in a flexed attitude. After dislodging the breech if necessary, by pushing above the pubic symphysis (never vaginally, which is culturally not acceptable), she crosses her hands over the woman's abdomen, positioning one on the baby's head, the other on the breech. Then, with very slow and careful pressure on head and breech, she "walks" the baby in the desired direction, in the course of which her hands become uncrossed. If she encounters resistance in one direction, she will try the reverse, but she emphasizes that the practitioner should never apply force. She does most versions in the 8th month but will continue her efforts up to and including labor.

We have neither seen complications nor heard stories about problems after ECV. The midwife herself recounts two cases of transient vaginal spotting, which had no further consequences. In the 10 years that we have worked in the area, there have been no breech births among her clients. Since she does about 100 deliveries a year, in a population of high-parity women, one would expect her to have had about 40 breech deliveries during that time.

For Yucatecan women, as for women in many traditional communities, ECV is the standard expected method for dealing with malpresentations. Version is seen as clearly beneficial for mother and child, and stories about the benefits and unproblematical nature of the procedure are easily elicited. Our observations suggest that to the extent that ECV is successful in Yucatan (and maybe in other traditional societies as well), this success may be predicated on the midwife's extraordinary skill and extensive experience in palpation and manipulation, aided by the fact that she works with a fetus and maternal body with which she is intimately familiar. On the woman's part, we note complete relaxation, which is possible in her own hut, in the presence of supportive and experienced family members. And finally, we might consider that the culturally conditioned expectation that turning the baby is the right thing to do, a procedure which is done routinely and without problems, may itself contribute to the positive outcome.

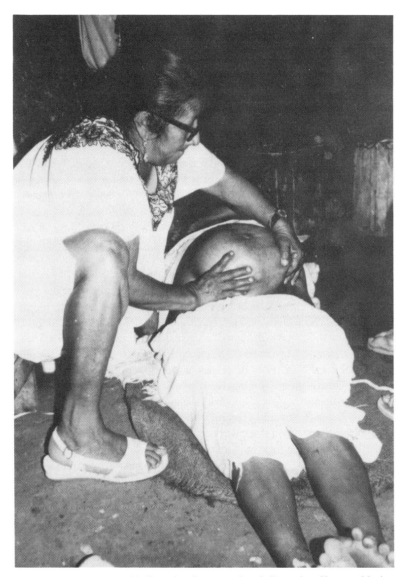

FIGURE 1. Maya Indian midwife performing external cephalic version, Yucatan, Mexico. (Courtesy, Brigitte Jordan and Nancy Fuller.)

The Conventional Medical Approach to ECV

ECV, as it was performed routinely by medical practitioners in the United States and still is by physicians and trained midwives in many other countries, utilizes the same basic technique as that used by traditional birth attendants. The major differences are the transfer of the procedure from the woman's territory to the physician's office or clinic and the addition of a simple technological aid for monitoring the fetal heart, the stethoscope. In addition, some conventional practitioners have used anesthesia to effect a more complete relaxation of the uterus. There exists a rich body of literature on conventional ECV in medical journals, obstetrical texts, and midwifery handbooks worldwide, probably containing reports on close to 10,000 cases.

Before a version is attempted, the woman's bladder and rectum should be empty. She lies on her back on a flat table with a pillow under her shoulders and knees. This permits slight flexion of the body, taking tension off the abdominal muscles and making her more comfortable and relaxed. After determining the position of the fetus, usually by palpation and more recently by ultrasound, and ascertaining the fetal heart rate by auscultation, the first step is to gently disengage the breech if it has descended into the pelvis. Facing the woman's feet, the operator lifts the breech out of the pelvis either with both hands or by sliding one hand abdominally between the maternal symphysis and the fetal breech. If disengagement is difficult, the foot of the table may be raised. Some practitioners find the Trendelenburg position helpful, and others will attempt a vaginal displacement. Once the breech has been dislodged, one hand of the operator then pushes the head, the other the breech, and by a series of pushes and/or taps on breech and head the fetus is gradually guided to a transverse position. The most difficult part may be negotiating the narrow diameter of the uterus, but after that a slight push is often all that is needed to complete the version. Sometimes uterine contractions start up, and in that case one should maintain the progress achieved so far by holding the fetus in place and then proceed again when the uterus relaxes. In no case should force be exerted against a contracted uterus. Finally, the fetal heart rate is again ascertained, and in the rare case that it should not normalize quickly (suggesting a short cord or cord entanglement), the fetus is returned to its original position.

Some practitioners advocate auscultating the fetal heart at various times throughout the procedure, possibly with the aid of a head stethoscope.[31] Conventional practitioners tend to consider the cooperation of the woman essential and suggest that a proper explanation of the procedure and its potential benefits is conducive to gaining the mother's cooperation and sincere efforts at relaxation. Pain is rarely mentioned but is considered an indication for abandoning the attempt for the time being and trying again in a few days.

The underlying idea in version is to maintain, or produce, flexion of the fetal body, making it as nearly ovoid in shape as possible. Usually, this is best accomplished by turning the fetus forward in the direction of the small parts, that is, with the head leading, although if that does not work, turning in the opposite direction is sometimes advocated.[6,13,23] Failure to achieve flexion is often associated with frank breech presentation with extended legs, which may splint the fetal trunk and head so effectively that it is impossible to get the fetal back to curve.

A common concern among conventional practitioners is the application of too much force. Although a few of them have used anesthesia on occasion when simple version failed,[12,33] there is general agreement that damage to the placenta is most likely to occur when the manipulations of the operator are not held in check by the subjective feelings of an anesthetized patient.[5,23,31,35] Extensive use of anesthesia seems never to have caught on in the United States, but studies from Scotland[2] and Ireland[28] indicate that the risks of ECV are higher with anesthesia. Apart from direct effects of the anesthetic, the more vigorous manipulation apparently increases the incidence of premature labor and placental abruption. Another study shows that for versions done under anesthesia, the fetal mortality is about four times as high as when no anesthesia is employed and the incidence of vaginal bleeding is substantially greater and more severe.[35]

It was noted earlier that many investigators report no fetal mortality attributable to conventional ECV.[13,20,31,33,35] In situations where mortality does occur, it is in every case a mere fraction of the expected breech mortality.[6,12,35,37] The incidence of complications such as premature separation of the placenta or fetal distress is similarly low, but some degree of suspicion about accuracy of reporting is raised when one realizes that the reported frequency is often much less than what would be expected in a normal obstetrical population. One report, for example, finds only 2 cases of prepartum bleeding in a review of more than 2,000 cases of version without anesthesia,[35] whereas *Williams Obstetrics*[30] cites an incidence of once in every 55 to 150 pregnancies.

In the face of enthusiastic and almost uniform advocacy of ECV by conventional practitioners, the literature is rather devoid of critics who present data. There is one important exception. Bradley-Watson[3] reports that in a group of 866 English version patients there were 8 intrauterine deaths within 24 hours of the procedure (0.9%), a 3% antepartum hemorrhage rate, 1.2% premature labor, and 0.6% premature rupturing of membranes, for a total complication rate of 4.4%. (Some women had more than one complication.) He points out that in the presence of a liberal cesarean section policy which lets only favorable cases come to breech delivery, the perinatal loss in modern, well-equipped institutions is rarely as high as 1%. He therefore concludes that in modern obstetrical practice a policy of routine version has decreasing value. His negative conclusion is based on the high fetal mortality he encountered. One cannot help but note the discrepancy in outcomes between Bradley-Watson's series of 866 version patients with 8 fetal deaths attributed to ECV, and the American series of Ranney, with 0 deaths in 860 patients. With such wide disparity in outcomes, great caution must be exercised in basing advocacy or condemnation of ECV on single studies.

The philosophy underlying conventional ECV is little different from that of the traditional approach. Version is seen not so much as an obstetrical intervention but as a way to give nature a helping hand in accomplishing what it intends to accomplish. Practiced by manipulatively skilled individuals as a "gentle art," ECV is considered by conventional practitioners to be a benign and fairly riskless procedure—an attitude for which the majority of outcome reports provides justification.

The Tocolytic Approach to ECV

In the last few years, mostly in Europe[7,18,19,27,34] but also in the United States,[38] ECV has appeared in a new form: It is performed with the aid of tocolytic (uterine relaxant) drugs, either alone or in combination with anesthesia, sedatives, or analgesics, and supported by ultrasound and external electronic fetal heart monitoring. This type of version is usually done very close to term, typically after the 37th week, under conditions where an immediate cesarean section can be performed should complications arise. ECV at this late date has some definite advantages: Most unnecessary versions are avoided; the fetus, once turned, is unlikely to revert; and if serious complications should occur, a cesarean section can be performed on a hopefully mature baby. On the negative side, one might consider the transformation of ECV into a thoroughly medicalized, technologized, drug-supported, in-hospital procedure. Most importantly, however, there exists the possibility that the complication rate is higher than with "gentle version," since tocolysis and a less than fully conscious patient allow the application of the greater force necessary with less amniotic fluid and a larger fetus. It should be noted that the total number of tocolytic versions reported in the literature so far is less than 500, so that outcome figures must be viewed with extreme caution.

The pharmacological agents that effect uterine relaxation during version are the same as those used to inhibit premature labor: primarily terbutaline sulfate (Bricanyl), fenoterol (Partusisten), which is commonly used in Europe, and, more recently, ritodrine hydrochloride (Yutopar),[38] given intravenously. Isoxsuprine administered by intramuscular injection was used in a Finnish study,[40] but it was employed only as an occasional adjunct to what was otherwise a conventional approach to ECV.

Before tocolytic version is attempted, a detailed ultrasound study determines fetal lie, presentation, attitude, estimated weight, placental location, and amount of amniotic fluid. In some institutions a nonstress test is performed and reactivity is established. The fetal heart rate is monitored for about an hour before the procedure is begun. Venous blood is drawn for Kleihauer-Betke (K-B) analysis, electrolytes, and glucose. An intravenous line is started. The maternal heart rate is continuously monitored electronically, and maternal blood pressure is recorded every 5 minutes, since cardiovascular disturbances and dropping blood pressure have been reported as side effects of the beta-mimetic tocolytic drugs.[11]

For the version, the woman lies on a flat table, her legs somewhat bent, slightly turned toward her side, since cardiovascular side effects may be enhanced by compression of the vena cava. In cases where full intubation anesthesia is used (with the intent of finishing up with a cesarean section if the version fails), the woman is in the lithotomy position in an operating room.[19] The tocolytic agent is then infused for 10 to 15 minutes prior to the version attempt and maintained until completion, often accompanied by sedation, analgesics, or anesthesia. When a sufficient depth of relaxation is reached, the breech is pushed out of the pelvis either externally or vaginally, possibly by an assistant, and then the operator pushes the fetal head in a *backward* direction without handling the breech. This method, initiated by Saling and Muller-Holve in Germany,[27,34] results in a "backward flip" of the fetus, and only if this fails to work is the forward turn attempted. Mechanically, ECV under tocolysis is thus the opposite of the traditional and conventional version procedure, in which the operator manipulates breech and head at the same time and usually in a forward direction.

During the version the fetal heart rate is auscultated several times or possibly kept under surveillance with both real-time ultrasound B-scanning and fetal heart rate monitoring (Doppler ultrasound).[38] Monitoring is continued afterward, typically for an hour or until a reactive nonstress test reappears. The procedure is interrupted if the discomfort becomes intolerable to the patient or if fetal heart rate decelerations are noted. Once the fetus is turned, success is documented by ultrasound if palpation leaves any doubt.

Venous blood for K-B analysis is again obtained 30 minutes after the version, and for Rh-negative patients, one more in 24 hours. In case fetomaternal transfusion is detected, gamma globulin is administered.

Because of the small number of studies, plagued by extremely small sample sizes and inconsistent reporting, the outcome data for tocolytic ECV are even less adequate than those for the conventional medical approach. Nevertheless, again with a single exception, reported outcome data are positive. There is some evidence that tocolytic version decreases fetal risk, since a significant improvement in the clinical and acidotic status of turned newborns has been reported.[34] No fetal mortality has been attributed to tocolytic ECV, but it appears that serious complications such as placental damage and fetal distress are more common than with the conventional gentle version.[18,19,34] There is also a higher incidence of fetomaternal hemorrhage and of metabolic and cardiovascular side effects,[19,24,34,38] which are reported generally to disappear with cessation of manipulation or assumption of the lateral position by the woman. Serious complications are routinely resolved by cesarean section, in an environment where surgery tends to be the rule for breech presentation anyway. Under such circumstances, the impact of ECV on the cesarean section rate is pronounced—a result that is reported by all investigators.

The single study which arrives at negative conclusions comes from Germany. Lehmann and co-workers,[19] who were able to turn only 27 of 51 (53%) of the fetuses, report 3 emergency cesareans (2 of these for partial premature separation of the placenta); 4 massive fetomaternal hemorrhages; and no significant improvements in pH-value and Apgar scores of the turned newborns. Without taking the positive outcomes of others into account, they conclude that in view of their low success rate and high incidence of complications, tocolytic ECV cannot be recommended.

With the tocolytic method, ECV has become an obstetrical intervention that relies for its proper execution on the resources of modern high-technology obstetrics. It appears particularly attractive in an environment where breeches are liberally or generally managed by cesarean. Given the scanty data reported in the literature, an objective, data-based assessment of the method is not possible at this time. If further tocolytic studies produce results that are consistent with the majority of presently available outcome figures, tocolytic ECV may represent a reasonable alternative to routine cesarean section. Nevertheless, reasoning as much from the nature of the procedure as from the data, one might want to be concerned about problems in three areas: placental separation or abruption caused by the application of too much force; similarly caused fetomaternal hemorrhage; and cardiovascular side effects due to drug administration.

Summary Assessment of ECV

A review of the biomedical literature on ECV makes clear that the data for an objective assessment of the risks and benefits of version simply do not exist yet. At the same time, there are indications that a purely biomedical framework may not be sufficient for answering all of the questions. Observation of the procedure in various settings suggests that it is *not* robust across individual practitioners, professional support structures, or cultural expectations; but there exist no studies which acknowledge such variables, much less incorporate them in any research design. One may suspect that the biomedical framework within which ECV has been investigated leads us to look at a narrow set of variables which provide only a partial answer to the question of success and failure of ECV. Psychosocial and cultural factors may explain the remainder.

Biomedical data do not allow the argument that ECV is either superior or inferior to the standard management options. But if we dispense with the pretense of arguing from scientific data for a moment and admit commonsensical reasoning, it would appear that ECV provides an attractive alternative. When successful, version will save some proportion of babies from breech or abdominal delivery. And when it fails, the standard options are still available. However, the "facts" here do not speak for themselves, and rational people have come down on opposite sides of the issues.

ECV dropped out of the American system during a time period which also saw increased emphasis on "active management" of labor, a rise in obstetrical interventions, and a growing reliance on pharmacology, technology, and surgery. Within this environment, cesarean section emerged as the standard solution to the problem of breech presentation, whereas alternative solutions became suspect by practitioners and clients alike. There arose a consensual culture of birth whose justification is conducted in the language of biomedicine while its practices are rooted in ideology and history. In the last analysis, we may be dealing here with a set of issues that lie where the science of medicine shades into the culture of doctoring.

REFERENCES

1. Banta HD, Thacker SB. *Costs and benefits of electronic fetal monitoring: A review of the literature*. National Center for Health Services Research, Washington, DC, Publication no. (PHS) 79–3245, US Department of Health, Education, and Welfare, 1979.

2. Bonnar J, Howie PW, MacLennon H. External cephalic version with anesthesia. *JAMA* 205:97–101, 1968.

3. Bradley-Watson PJ. The decreasing value of external cephalic version in modern obstetric practice. *Am J Obstet Gynecol* 123:237–240, 1975.

4. Brenner, WE, Bruce RD, Hendricks CH. The characteristics and perils of breech presentation. *Am J Obstet Gynecol* 118:700, 1974.

5. Dexeus FS, Dexeus T de B. *Tratado de obstetricia.* Tomo II. Barcelona, Salvat Editores, 1957.

6. Donovan HCE. Antenatal treatment of breech presentation. *Med J Aust*, II:617–621, 1932.

7. Fall O, Nilsson BA. External cephalic version in breech presentation under tocolysis. *Obstet Gynecol* 53:712–715, 1979.

8. Fischer-Rasmussen W, Trolle D. Abdominal versus vaginal delivery in breech presentation. *Acta Obstet Gynecol Scand* 46:69–76, 1967.

9. Fuller N, Jordan B. *Turning the baby (external cephalic version–Maya Indians of Yucatan)*, ¾'' cassette videotape, 1979.

10. Fuller N, Jordan B. Maya women and the end of the birthing period: Postpartum massage-and-binding in Yucatan, Mexico. *Med Anthropol* 5:35–50, 1981.

11. Gerris J, Thiery M, Bogaert M, et al. Randomized trial of two beta-mimetic drugs (ritodrine and fenoterol) in acute intra-partum tocolysis. *Europ J Clin Pharmacol* 18:443–448, 1980.

12. Gibberd GF. An investigation into the results of breech labour, and of prophylactic external cephalic version during pregnancy; with a note on the technique of external version. *J Obstet Gynaecol Br Emp* 34:509–519, 1927.

13. Glassman O. The use of external cephalic version in an outdoor maternity clinic. *Am J Obstet Gynecol* 24:277–278, 1932.

14. Hall JE, Kohl SG, O'Brien F, et al. Breech presentation and perinatal mortality. *Am J Obstet Gynecol* 91:665, 1965.

15. Hibbard LT, Schumann WR. Prophylactic external cephalic version in an obstetric practice. *Am J Obstet Gynecol* 116:511–518, 1973.

16. Jordan B. *Birth in four cultures: A crosscultural investigation of childbirth in Yucatan, Holland, Sweden and the United States.* Montreal, Eden Press Women's Publications, 1978.

17. Kay MA (ed). *The anthropology of human birth.* Philadelphia, FA Davis Co, 1982.

18. Kyank HR, Severin W, Stranz G. Preventive version of breech presentation—first results and complications. *Zentralbl Gynaekol* 99:1008–1013, 1977.

19. Lehmann V, Hodt C, Criegern T. External version from breech to vertex presentation. *Z Geburtsh U Perinat* 181:390–395, 1977.

20. MacArthur JL. Reduction of the hazards of breech presentation by external cephalic version. *Am J Obstet Gynecol* 88:302–306, 1968.

21. Marcus RG, Crewe-Brown H, Krawitz S, et al. Feto-maternal haemorrhage following successful and unsuccessful attempts at external cephalic version. *Br J Obstet Gynaecol* 82:578–580, 1975.

22. Marieskind H. *An evaluation of caesarean section in the United States.* Washington, DC, US Department of Health, Education, and Welfare, 1979.

23. McGuinness FG. Prophylactic external cephalic version in breech presentation. *Canad Med Assoc J* 18:289–292, 1928.

24. Meyenburg M, Busch W. Die äussere Wendung unter Einsatz der Tocolyse. *Z Geburtsh Perinatol* 180:427, 1976.

25. Minkoff HL, Schwartz RH. The rising cesarean section rate: Can it safely be reversed? *Obstet Gynecol* 56:135–143, 1980.

26. Morgan HS, Kane SH. An analysis of 16,327 breech births. *JAMA* 187:262–264, 1964.

27. Muller-Holve W, Saling E. Tocolysis for external version of breech presentation close to term. *Z Geburtsh U Perinatol* 179:24–29, 1975.

28. Neely MR. External cephalic version under anesthesia. *J Obstet Gynaecol Br Commonw* 68:490–497, 1961.

29. Newell JL. Prophylactic external cephalic version. *Am J Obstet Gynecol* 42:256–261, 1941.

30. Pritchard J, MacDonald PC. *Williams Obstetrics*. New York, Appleton-Century-Crofts, 1976.

31. Ranney B. The gentle art of external cephalic version. *Am J Obstet Gynecol* 116:239–251, 1973.

32. Rovinsky JJ, Miller JA, Kaplan S. Management of breech presentation at term. *Am J Obstet Gynecol* 115:497–513, 1973.

33. Ryder GH. Breech presentations treated by cephalic versions in the consecutive deliveries of 1,700 women. *Am J Obstet Gynecol* 45:1004–1025, 1943.

34. Saling E, Muller-Holve W. External cephalic version under tocolysis. *J Perinat Med* 3:115–122, 1975.

35. Siegel TA, McNally HB. Breech presentations and prophylactic external cephalic version. *Am J Obstet Gynecol* 37:86–93, 1939.

36. Stevenson CS. Certain concepts in the handling of breech and transverse presentations in late pregnancy. *Am J Obstet Gynecol* 62:488–505, 1951.

37. Trubkowitch MV, Archangelsky BA. Results of external prophylactic version, *Br Med J* 1:220, 1944.

38. Van Dorsten JP, Schifrin BS, Wallace RL. Randomized control trial of external cephalic version with tocolysis in late pregnancy. *Am J Obstet Gynecol* 141:417–424, 1981.

39. Young D, Mahan C. *Unnecessary cesareans: Ways to avoid them*. Minneapolis, International Childbirth Education Association, 1980.

40. Ylikorkala O, Hartikainen-Sorri AL. Value of external version in fetal malpresentation in combination with the use of ultrasound. *Acta Obstet Gynecol Scand* 56:63–67, 1977.

SUBMITTED: AUGUST, 1982
ACCEPTED· AUGUST, 1982

AMNIOTOMY

Penelope P. Simkin

Although amniotomy (artificial rupture of the membranes) is a common, even routine procedure in many obstetrical practices, the question of its appropriateness and efficacy is rarely addressed in leading obstetrical textbooks.[1-4] There is, however, a large body of literature covering the subject. Usually considered a minor procedure, amniotomy is performed for the following reasons: to induce labor; to augment labor; to allow placement of a scalp electrode and intrauterine pressure catheter for internal electronic fetal monitoring; or to inspect amniotic fluid for the presence of meconium.

The procedure is carried out after a check of fetal heart tones and sterile vaginal examination to determine the station and condition of the cervix. The physician or midwife may first ''strip'' the membranes; that is, he or she inserts a finger through the soft dilatable cervix and separates the membranes from the lower uterine segment. Then, using a finger or an amnioscope as a guide, the practitioner inserts a membrane hook or other instrument, catches and tears the membranes. Usually a gush or at least a trickle of fluid follows. Contraindications to amniotomy include a high presenting part, presentation other than vertex, an unripe cervix, or abnormal fetal heart rate patterns.[5]

Spontaneous Rupture of the Membranes

Amniotomy either to start or to hasten labor represents a significant intervention and modification of the physiological process. Spontaneous rupture of the membranes before labor begins occurs only about 10% to 12% of the time (20% of those are preterm; the remainder are at term).[6] Caldeyro-Barcia and co-workers found that when labor begins with the membranes intact, 66% remain intact at least until the cervix is fully dilated. In fact, in 12% of cases the bag of waters is still intact at delivery.[7]

Benefits of Intact Membranes

Does the bag of waters provide some benefit to mother or fetus? Intact membranes provide some protection against infection, both through the intrinsic opsonic and antimicrobial properties of amniotic fluid[8] and as a barrier to outside sources of infection. When membranes are ruptured, either artificially or spontaneously, both forms of protection are lost, increasing the likelihood of infection and conferring a sense of urgency and a time limit for delivery. In addition, amniotic fluid is a source of liquid and possibly some nourishment for the fetus, who swallows it frequently; it provides an environment of stable temperature; it collects fetal excretions; it protects the fetus from direct trauma; and through its constant lubrication of the fetus and other intrauterine contents, allows freedom of fetal movement.[9]

Other forms of protection afforded by intact membranes will be discussed in the following sections of this chapter, which will include a review of the literature as it applies to amniotomy for the purposes of induction and/or augmentation of labor, and brief discussion of other purposes of amniotomy.

Amniotomy to Induce Labor

The general subject of induction of labor, with its risks and benefits, is covered elsewhere in this book. In this chapter, one specific form of labor induction will be discussed—amniotomy.

When the cervix and station have been evaluated for inducibility and given high scores (see Bishop Pelvic Scoring System, Table 1), the likelihood of success in initiating labor approaches 90%.[10]

Risks of Amniotomy

The lower the Bishop score, the less the chance of success with amniotomy and the more desirable are pharmacological means of induction, such as oxytocin infusion or the use of prostaglandins. Prostaglandins are in widespread use in Europe for ripening the cervix and inducing labor, but they have not yet been approved for such uses in the United States. If am-

TABLE 1	PELVIC SCORING SYSTEM (BISHOP SCORE)*			
FACTOR	SCORE: 0	1	2	3
Station (Presenting Part)	-3	-2	-1,0	+1,+2
Cervical Dilatation	0 cm	1-2 cm	3-4 cm	5-6 cm
Cervical Effacement	0-30%	40-50%	60-70%	80%
Cervical Consistency	Firm	Medium	Soft	----
Cervical Position	Posterior	Middle	Anterior	----

*Modified from Bishop EH: Obstet Gynecol 24:266, 1964.[11]

niotomy alone does not bring on labor within a short time, oxytocin will be initiated to hasten the process.

Sellers and co-workers offer another explanation for the failure of amniotomy to induce labor in some women while succeeding in others.[12] In their study of 16 women following amniotomy at term, 7 women were in established labor within 5½ hours; the remaining 9 required oxytocin. The PGFM (the major circulating metabolite of prostaglandin F) levels were measured in all women. There was an initial rise in all 16 women within 5 minutes after amniotomy, but only in the group where amniotomy was successful was there a continuing and sustained rise in PGFM levels. The two groups did not differ in Bishop scores, age, birth weight, or gestation. The clinical implications of this study are not yet clear, but it does indicate a "readiness" for labor in some subjects, and a lack of readiness in others, which is unrelated to the more familiar clinical signs of readiness for induction.

Besides the fact that amniotomy for induction carries a 10% possibility of failure, even with careful patient selection, there are other risks to mother and baby. The principal drawback to amniotomy is the possibility of infection ascending to the fetus and uterus. The longer the membranes are ruptured and the more often the mother is examined vaginally, the greater the likelihood of infection.[13] Therefore, whether rupture of the membranes before labor is spontaneous or artificial, it is extremely important to limit vaginal examinations and to use scrupulous sterile technique when performing the examination. In addition, once rupture of the membranes at term has occurred, the mother might be motivated to use physiological means to bring on labor if she and her attendants wish to avoid oxytocin induction. Breast stimulation, either by the mother herself or lovingly by her partner, or even by suckling a borrowed baby in an atmosphere of privacy and calm, may be all that is needed to initiate effective labor contractions. Jhirad and Vago reported breast stimulation to be effective in initiating labor in 69.6% of the 204 women studied.[14] Oxytocin is released by the mother's pituitary gland when the breasts are stimulated, causing uterine contractions which are frequently sufficient to initiate labor.

Other methods of bringing on labor— castor oil, enemas, herbal teas, walking—are also utilized with inconsistent results. These methods are usually left to the discretion of the woman. Not having been subjected to scientific investigation, they are relegated to the "home remedy" category, that is, considered as generally harmless and with some anecdotal evidence of efficacy.

Besides the risk of infection, the risk of prolapsed cord exists, especially if the presenting part is not engaged. Even when the presenting part is well applied to the cervix, there remains an incidence of prolapsed cord of about 1 in 2,000 apparently normal cases.[15] Although the risk is small, it deserves careful consideration in balancing benefits of amniotomy against risks. In an effort to reduce the risks of prolapsed cord, even in normal cases, it might be wise to conduct a vaginal examination while the woman is upright. If the head is engaged or well applied to the cervix when the woman is upright, the chances of prolapsed cord while she stands or walks are extremely slim. Sometimes as the woman assumes the erect position, the fetal head will descend and engage. In that case the upright position would be beneficial in avoiding prolapsed cord.[15]

Other potential risks to the fetus have been discovered by Caldeyro-Barcia and co-workers as a result of the Latin American Collaborative Study of 1,124 labors in a prospective randomized trial.[7] Only women meeting the following criteria were included: healthy term pregnancies; no cephalopelvic disproportion; spontaneous labors; no medication during labor; intact membranes; less than 5 cm dilated; and ending with spontaneous vaginal deliveries. Every other woman had her membranes ruptured artificially at 4 to 5 cm. Membranes were allowed to rupture spontaneously in the remaining women. The two groups were compared for effects of amniotomy on the labors and the fetuses.

The study found important risks associated with amniotomy, chiefly due to uneven distribution of pressure during uterine contractions. There was an increased likelihood of caput succedaneum (edematous swelling on the fetal scalp due to pressures to which the head is subjected during labor); excessive molding of the fetal head; higher incidence of Type 1 dips (early decelerations) in the fetal heart rate; occlusion of the fetal umbilical vessels; and indications of poorer fetal oxygenation.

When the membranes are intact, hydrostatic pressure is more evenly distributed over the fetus, placenta, cord, and presenting part, with counterpressure from the forewaters providing some protection of the fetal scalp against caput succedaneum and disalignment of cranial bones in cephalic presentations. When membranes are ruptured, a greater proportion of the pressure of the contractions is accepted by the fetal head, causing elongation of the head, caput succedaneum, and possible excessive bone disalignment. Although such effects are also seen with intact membranes, they are more frequent and more pronounced when membranes are ruptured early. Forty-four percent of neonates in the early amniotomy group as opposed to 35% in the late rupture group showed disalignment of cranial bones, a statistically significant difference in this study sample from which cases of cephalopelvic disproportion (an important cause of disalignment of cranial bones) were excluded. Thirty-four percent of neonates in the early amniotomy group had caput succedaneum. The later in labor that spontaneous rupture occurred, the lower the incidence of caput succedaneum. In the group of 61 women whose membranes remained intact until delivery, the prevalence of caput succedaneum fell to 5%. Although caput succedaneum is not in itself considered harmful, if combined with greater molding of the fetal head, it may indicate that without the protection of the bag of waters, the fetal head endures significantly more pressure than when the membranes are intact. In occasional difficult births, the presence of the bag of waters could conceivably afford enough protection to prevent subdural hemorrhage or other cerebral lesions. Caldeyro-Barcia cited studies[16-18] showing positive associations between both encephalic lesions seen on autopsy and incidence of mental retardation, and the number of hours elapsing between rupture of the membranes and birth.

Amniotomy was also associated with a higher incidence of Type 1 dips. Type 1 dips are caused by three factors: (1) compression of the fetal head which increases when the membranes are ruptured; (2) engagement of the fetal head below 0 station, explaining the frequently observed Type 1 dips observed during late second stage; and (3) occlusion of umbilical vessels during contractions.

In the Latin American study reported by Caldeyro-Barcia and co-workers, the percentage of contractions with Type 1 dips before engagement of the fetal head was almost four times higher in the early amniotomy group than in the late rupture group (15.62% versus 4.39%). After engagement the protective quality of intact membranes was even more evident, although the incidence of Type 1 dips increased for both groups (45.68% for the early amniotomy group compared with 9.24% in the group with intact membranes).

The cord occlusion associated with absence of amniotic fluid postulated by Caldeyro-Barcia and co-workers was confirmed in monkey studies by Gabbe and associates.[19] When amniotic fluid was removed from the uteri of pregnant monkeys, there were variable heart rate decelerations which returned to normal patterns when the fluid was replaced. They concluded that cord compression leading to decelerations occurred when the fluid was absent.

Steer and co-workers studied the effect of membrane rupture on fetal heart rate in induced labors and found significant increases in the incidence of fetal heart rate decelerations in a group with early amniotomy compared with a group in which the membranes ruptured spontaneously.[20] In the latter group, the decelerations were not present until spontaneous rupture occurred in the last hour of labor. Decelerations were either Type 1 (early decelerations) or Type 3 (variable decelerations). This study confirmed the findings of Caldeyro-Barcia's study described earlier. The authors, however, pointed out that all 20 babies, including the 12 in the earlier amniotomy group, were in "excellent condition" as measured only by Apgar scores. From this they drew the conclusion that the early amniotomy group was "not subjected to any serious form of stress." They did not report on any other aspects of the infants' condition, such as head molding and disalignment of cranial bones. They believe, as do many others, that the presumed advantage of early amniotomy, namely shortening labor, outweighs the theoretical risks accompanying increased incidence of fetal heart rate decelerations. The problem with this conclusion is that the sample size (20 subjects) for the study was too small to draw such an inference.

In an effort to replicate the work of Caldeyro-Barcia and his group, Baumgarten used a similar protocol to that of the Latin American study in a smaller study of 165 gravidas (94 with spontaneous onset of labor and 71 with induced labor).[21] His findings generally agreed with the findings of Caldeyro-Barcia's group. They found more Type 1 dips, more caput succedaneum, shorter labors, and no difference in Apgar scores or neurological assessment at age 24 and 48 hours in the early amniotomy group when compared with a late spontaneous rupture group.

Another group of investigators, Martell and colleagues, studied acid-base balance and cord blood gas values in 21 infants of mothers who had early amniotomy in labor and in 17 infants of mothers whose membranes remained intact until second stage.[23] All pregnancies in the study were low-risk. The pH of umbilical venous blood was higher in the late rupture group (median = 7.36) than in the early amniotomy group (median = 7.30; $p<0.01$). The pH of umbilical arterial blood followed the same trend (7.31 versus 7.25; $p<0.025$). The PCO_2 in umbilical venous blood was less and hemoglobin saturation greater in the late rupture group ($p<0.05$). All these results are evidence of better uteroplacental circulation in the late rupture group. Although none of the blood values or fetal monitoring records indicated fetal distress, when the authors compared their findings with other analyses of acid-base balance in umbilical vessels, they found that median values of both pH and PO_2 in the late spontaneous rupture group were well above the averages reported by most authors; their PCO_2 values were the lowest recorded. Status of the membranes had not been considered in the other studies. The authors concluded that in low-risk pregnancies, ". . . when amniotic membranes remain intact at least until full dilatation, the infant is more likely to be born with a 'better acid-base balance' . . . This observation may be even more important in high-risk pregnancies where the utero-placental circulation is compromised.''

The point by Martell and group is worth emphasizing. If significant increases in the incidence of Type 1 and Type 3 dips, umbilical cord occlusion, cranial bone disalignment, caput succedaneum, and lower umbilical vessel pH and PO_2 values are associated with early amniotomy in low-risk pregnancies, then one may conclude that fetal reserves are being depleted simply by this procedure. The effects on a healthy neonate are unremarkable, but in a questionable or clearly high-risk situation, refraining from the use of this procedure might improve infant outcome. The need for further research in this area is obvious.

Amniotomy clearly causes measurable deviations from the physiological course of labor, which under some circumstances may be detrimental to infant outcome. For this reason, if considering amniotomy either for induction or augmentation of labor, one should be very certain that the potential benefits outweigh the potential risks. The benefit usually claimed for amniotomy is that it shortens labor. Even this claim, however, is subject to vigorous disagreement from at least one prominent investigator.[10]

In Friedman's review of the literature and discussion of his own extensive work on amniotomy, he concludes that labors following amniotomy do not differ from labors of spontaneous onset in terms of labor progress, if matched ''case-for-case according to pre-labor status of the cervix.''[23] This claim stands out against the many studies indicating that amniotomy speeds labor.[20,21,24–26] These studies, however, only compared lengths of labor in two groups of patients: early amniotomy and late rupture groups. All these studies, except that of Schwarcz and co-workers,[25] involved small numbers of subjects. Schwarcz's study involved 1,413 labors in which alternate women had their membranes ruptured. Their labors were, on the average, 50 minutes shorter than those in which the membranes were not ruptured artificially.

Friedman's approach differed. Using objective criteria and a large study population, he recorded Bishop scores of prelabor state of the cervix and charted labor progress (dilatation and descent) and all interventions, including amniotomy, against time. Thus he was able to observe the causal and time relationship between the intervention and labor progress. Using this method with a large study population, he concluded that whereas amniotomy is effective in initiating labor in patients with high Bishop scores, it made no measurable difference in labor progress when compared to patients with similar Bishop scores who did not have amniotomies.

Even if labor could be shortened by amniotomy, would the shorter labor be beneficial to the outcome? Philpott and Castle concluded from their study that shorter labors are associated with lower fetal and maternal morbidity than longer ones.[27] O'Driscoll and colleagues, in two separate studies,[28,29] suggested that active management (including amniotomy and oxytocin) be widely utilized to assure that no labor exceed 12 hours—the "ideal" limit.

Caldeyro-Barcia and co-workers[16] do not agree that shorter labors are safer; they may even be associated with poorer outcomes for infants. They cite Niswander and Gordon's work,[30] indicating that both perinatal mortality and neurological abnormalities at one year of age increased when the duration of first stage decreased below an optimal range. Chalmers and colleagues, in their comparative evaluation of the outcomes of active and conservative management of labor, stated, "Our research suggests that if there are either beneficial or adverse effects on perinatal outcome of an active approach to induction and acceleration of labor. . ., then the effect is very small."[31]

Amniotomy to Speed Normal Labor

As Lynaugh explained in her review of early elective amniotomy,[32] "It is believed that amniotomy stimulates uterine action and thus stimulates labor." She points out that the practitioner waits until there is good evidence of true labor (strong regular contractions, 4 to 5 cm dilatation) before performing amniotomy in normal labor. The subsequent rapid dilatation usually seen is what one would correctly expect to happen in this active phase of labor. In a normal labor pattern there is always a rapid acceleration of dilatation at about 4 cm. Amniotomy is credited for progress that would have taken place anyway.

Amniotomy to Augment Prolonged Labor

Friedman systematically investigated and classified abnormal labor patterns,[24] examining the efficacy of amniotomy and other interventions in correcting or improving various prolonged labor patterns. Of the nine labor disorders defined by him (1–prolonged latent phase; 2–protracted active phase dilatation; 3–protracted descent; 4–prolonged deceleration phase; 5–secondary arrest of dilatation; 6–arrest of descent; 7–failure of descent; 8–precipitate dilatation; and 9–precipitate descent), amniotomy is widely utilized to attempt to correct the first six disorders. In prolonged latent phase, Friedman found that, at best, amniotomy was associated with prompt progress (defined as moving into the active phase within 3 hours after amniotomy) in less than 26.9% of the cases studied. At best, amniotomy was found to be "of dubious value" in improving a prolonged latent phase. Cardozo's group came to a similar conclusion in their study of active management of dysfunctional labors.[33] In all the other disorders, amniotomy was found to be "without effect in stimulating labor," "generally disappointing," or "entirely ineffectual." In the case of secondary arrest of dilatation, early amniotomy may sometimes even have caused the arrest. In 32% of the cases of secondary arrest of dilatation, there was no arrest until after the amniotomy. "Thus, there is an increasingly perplexing implication that amniotomy may be a retarding factor in dysfunctional labor...contrary to current opinion and widespread clinical impression and practice."[34]

Therefore, the evidence suggests that amniotomy may be of little or no benefit in augmenting labor, may adversely affect the condition of the fetus, and may expose both fetus and mother to additional risks of infection and cord prolapse.

Amniotomy for Detection of Meconium in the Fluid

It is frequently suggested that one benefit of amniotomy is that it allows the physician or midwife to detect meconium staining of the fluid—a sign of possible fetal distress.[1,35,36] One problem, of course, is that the procedure itself causes some reduction in fetal oxygenation due to added compression of the fetal head, and possibly the umbilical cord. If the fetus is already stressed, as would be indicated by the presence of meconium, the process of detecting it, in itself, would add to that stress. On the other hand, if the fetus is not stressed, it has to be delivered anyway because of the danger of infection presented by the amniotomy. As O'Driscoll and co-workers noted, "The release of a copious flow of clear liquor...presents a paradox, because the action that commits the patient to delivery shows that the fetus is not in danger..."[37]

A less invasive alternative was described by Saling[38] and by Benzie.[39] With amnioscopy, the fluid may be visualized through intact membranes. An endoscope with a light source is inserted through the partially dilated cervix and the fluid inspected through the translucent membranes. It is a procedure requiring training and experience to achieve reliability. Amnioscopy is not free from possible complications. If the cervix is closed, it may be impossible to pass the amnioscope. The membranes may rupture accidentally during the procedure. The amnioscope may introduce bacteria resulting in infection. Placenta previa, known or suspected, is an absolute contraindication to amnioscopy. These complications also exist with amniotomy.

Amnioscopy is not popular in the United States or Great Britain but is widely used in Europe.

The advantage of amnioscopy is that it is only diagnostic and, as such, assists in screening those who will require aggressive management. Amniotomy as a diagnostic procedure also introduces a potential risk factor to the labor. Aggressive management becomes necessary for many women having amniotomy, whether the fetus is doing well or not.

Amniotomy to Allow Placement of Fetal Scalp Electrode

Amniotomy is necessary if internal electronic fetal monitoring is indicated, to allow insertion of the fetal scalp electrode and the intrauterine pressure catheter. It is also a precursor to obtaining samples of fetal scalp blood for acid-base evaluation. Therefore, in high-risk situations, the use of amniotomy may be unavoidable. Once again, however, the practitioner is forced into a position where he or she must add to fetal stress in order to detect it.

Conclusion

Amniotomy is a widespread procedure whose value, except under some circumstances of high risk, is questionable at best. When the procedure has been subjected to careful scrutiny, possible risks have been discovered such as head and umbilical cord compression, resulting in possible excessive head molding and fetal distress. The assumed benefits of amniotomy in inducing labor, and particularly in augmenting labor, have not been proved in carefully controlled studies. In fact, objective evaluations of the procedure indicate little or no benefit in augmenting labor, and benefit in inducing labor only when the cervix is ripe and the presenting part engaged.

Without artificial rupture of the membranes, most labors will progress late into the first stage or beyond before spontaneous rupture occurs. The protection afforded by intact membranes should not be removed routinely through amniotomy.

REFERENCES

1. Pritchard JA, MacDonald PC: *Williams Obstetrics* (16th ed). New York, Appleton-Century-Crofts, 1980.

2. Garrey MM, Govan ADT, Hodge C, et al. *Obstetrics illustrated* (2nd ed). Edinburgh and London, 1974.

3. Walker J, MacGillivray I, MacNaughton MC. *Combined textbook of obstetrics and gynaecology.* (9th ed), Edinburgh, London, and New York, Churchill Livingstone, 1976.

4. Oxom H. *Oxorn-Foote: Human labor and birth* (4th ed). New York, Appleton-Century-Crofts, 1980.

5. Ibid, p. 588.

6. Ibid, p. 619.

7. Caldeyro-Barcia R, Schwarcz R, Belizan JM, et al. Adverse perinatal effects of early amniotomy during labor. In *Modern perinatal medicine*. Gluck L (ed). Chicago, Year Book Medical Publishers Inc., 1974.

8. Cone MJ, Steele RW, Marmer DJ, et al. Functional bacterial opsonic activity of human amniotic fluid. *Am J Obstet Gynecol* 142:282–287, 1982.

9. Jensen MD, Benson RC, Bobak IM. *Maternity care: The nurse and the family*. St Louis, CV Mosby Co, 1977, p 117.

10. Friedman EA. *Labor: Clinical evaluation and management* (2nd ed). New York, Appleton-Century-Crofts, 1978, pp 334–335.

11. Bishop EH. Pelvic scoring for elective induction. *Obstet Gynecol* 24:266–268, 1964.

12. Sellers SM, Mitchell MD, Anderson ABM, et al. The relation between the release of prostaglandins at amniotomy and the subsequent onset of labour. *Br J Obstet Gynaecol* 88:1211–1216, 1981.

13. Pritchard JA, MacDonald PC. op. cit. p 937; pp 408–410.

14. Jhirad A, Vago T. Induction of labor by breast stimulation. *Obstet Gynecol* 41:347–350, 1973.

15. Moore WMO. Antenatal care and the choice of place of birth. In *The place of birth*, Kitzinger S, Davis JA (eds). Oxford, New York, and Toronto, Oxford University Press, 1978.

16. Fedrick J, Butler NR. Certain causes of neonatal death. *Biol Neonate* 18:321–329, 1971.

17. Muller PF, Campbell HE, Graham WE, et al. Perinatal factors and their relationship to mental retardation and other parameters of development. *Am J Obstet Gynecol* 109:1205–1210, 1971.

18. Schwartz P. *Birth injuries of the newborn. Morphology, pathogenesis, clinical pathology, and prevention*. New York, Hafner Publishing Co, 1961.

19. Gabbe S, Ettinger B, Freeman R, et al. Umbilical cord compression associated with amniotomy: Laboratory observations. *Am J Obstet Gynecol* 126:353–355, 1976.

20. Steer PJ, Little DJ, Lewis NL, et al. The effect of membrane rupture on fetal heart rate in induced labour. *Br J Obstet Gynaecol* 83:454–459, 1976.

21. Baumgarten K. Advantages and disadvantages of low amniotomy. *J Perinat Med* 4:3–11, 1976.

22. Martell M, Belizan JM, Nieto F, et al. Blood acid-base balance at birth in neonates from labors with early and late rupture of membranes. *J Pediatr* 89:963–967, 1976.

23. Friedman EA. op cit. p 216.

24. Wetrich DW. Effect of amniotomy upon labor: A controlled study. *Obstet Gynecol* 35:800–806, 1970.

25. Schwarcz R, Diaz AG, Belizan JM, et al. Influence of amniotomy and maternal position on labor. In *Proceedings of the VIII World Congress of Gynecology and Obstetrics*. Amsterdam, Excerpta Medica, 1977.

26. Stewart P, Kennedy JH, Calder AA. Spontaneous labour: When should the membranes be ruptured? *Br J Obstet Gynaecol* 89:39–43, 1982.

27. Philpott RH, Castle WM. Cervicographs in the management of labour in primigravidae. *J Obstet Gynaecol Br Commonw* 79:592–602, 1972.

28. O'Driscoll K, Jackson RJA, Gallagher JT. Active management of labour and cephalopelvic disproportion. *J Obstet Gynaecol Br Commonw* 77:385–389, 1970.

29. O'Driscoll K, Stronge JM, Minogue M. Active management of labour. *Br Med J* 3:135–137, 1973.

30. Niswander KR, Gordon M. The women and their pregnancies. In *The Collaborative Perinatal Study of the National Institute of Neurological Diseases and Stroke*. Philadelphia, WB Saunders Co, 1972.

31. Chalmers I, Lawson JG, Turnbull AC. Evaluation of different approaches to obstetric care. Part II. *Br J Obstet Gynaecol* 83:930–933, 1976.

32. Lynaugh K. Effects of early elective amniotomy on the length of labor and the condition of the fetus. *J Nurs Midwifery* 25(4):3–9, 1980.

33. Cardozo LD, Gibb DMF, Studd JWW, et al. Predictive value of cervimetric labour patterns in primigravidae. *Br J Obstet Gynaecol* 89:33–38, 1982.

34. Friedman EA. op cit. p 105.

35. O'Driscoll K, Coughlan M, Fenton V, et al. Active management of labour: Care of the fetus. *Br Med J* 2:1451–1453, 1977.

36. Zuspan FP, Quilligan EJ. *Practical manual of obstetrical care*. St. Louis, CV Mosby Co, 1982, p 235.

37. O'Driscoll K, Carroll CJ, Coughlan M. Selective induction of labour. *Br Med J* 4:727–729, 1975.

38. Saling EZ, et al. The present situation of clinical monitoring of the fetus during labor. *J Perinat Med* 1:75, 1973.

39. Benzie RJ. Amniocentesis, amnioscopy, and fetoscopy. *Clin Obstet Gynecol* 7(3):439, 1980.

SUBMITTED: SEPTEMBER, 1982
ACCEPTED: SEPTEMBER, 1982

AN ASSESSMENT OF ELECTRONIC
FETAL MONITORING

Albert D. Haverkamp
Miriam Orleans

Electronic fetal monitoring (EFM) is an obstetrical technology that is now available in almost every obstetrical unit in the United States.[1,2] It has, however, become a controversial medical procedure. The controversy springs from varied medical as well as social concerns and has important implications for obstetrical practice.

First, the American attitude toward childbirth has increasingly, and in most cases appropriately, emphasized the "naturalness" of human reproduction. Thus any intervention in normal labor and delivery, whether with drugs, anesthesia, or technology, must be viewed with concern. Indeed, new concepts of maternal-infant bonding and family-centered childbirth have already produced many changes in standard obstetrical care. The new birthing areas in many hospitals and the interest in home delivery are signs of efforts to "normalize" the settings in which children are born.

Second, rising health care costs are a serious problem in the United States. New technologies in all areas of medical care have rapidly proliferated in the past three decades. Medical care each year claims an increasing share of the country's resources, and at the present writing about 10% of the Gross National Product is spent on health services in the United States. The contribution of increased technology to this high cost has been discussed by a number of economic and financial analysts.[3,4] The benefit of these technologies is not always well demonstrated, and studies of the benefit, effectiveness, efficiency, and cost of care are needed in all fields of practice, including obstetrics.

Third, American health care is under societal and professional pressure to improve maternal and infant health outcomes, as it becomes widely perceived that infant mortality in the United States is higher than that of other western nations. This record has, in fact, improved, even though other countries have been more successful. At the beginning of this century about 100 of every 1,000 infants born in the United States died before their first birth-

115

day. By 1979 infant mortality declined to 13 deaths per 1,000 live births.[5] Advances in neonatology, the development of regionalized perinatal networks, progress in the management of high-risk pregnant women, along with advances in newborn intensive care have all been viewed as beneficial, although the fraction of contribution of each of these factors to the decline in neonatal deaths is not yet clearly understood.

Because of its continuing concern with perinatal mortality, the obstetrical community has assumed a role of fetal advocacy. Thus increasingly complicated technologies such as EFM and fetal blood scalp (FBS) sampling combined with a more liberal use of cesarean sections have been viewed as efforts to reduce intrapartum deaths and neurological damage.

Finally, a new contractual relationship is developing between obstetrical professionals and their patients. Childbearing women are thought to be entitled to make decisions about their own health care. To do so, they must be provided with a reasonable amount of information about risks, benefits, and alternatives. Decisions about fetal monitoring potentially become a matter of patient choice rather than institutional policy. There are concerns that this choice will conflict with what the obstetrician feels are his or her ethical obligations to practice "good" medicine.

EFM Technology: What Does it Do?

Electronic fetal monitoring is based on the principle of continuously recording on polygraph the fetal heart rate (FHR) and the uterine contractions. Electronic fetal monitors are capable of obtaining these data indirectly (externally) or directly (internally).

Indirect (External) Fetal Heart Rate Monitoring

Indirect (external) monitoring is the most frequently used method. It has the advantage of being clinically uninvasive and may also be employed before the intrapartum period. The Doppler ultrasound technique is the most commonly used method of indirect fetal heart rate monitoring. The basic ultrasound transducer consists of a transmitting and receiving crystal. A jelly or mineral oil facilitates acoustical coupling between the transducer and the abdomen, and a belt holds the transducer in place. The transmitting crystal sends out a continuous acoustical wave. Any moving structures, such as the myocardial wall, valves of the fetal heart, or pulsating blood vessels, send the receiving crystal a signal in the form of a reflected wave, which changes in frequency. The Doppler device cannot measure beat-to-beat variability in fetal heart rates.

FHR determinations by Doppler ultrasound are relatively accurate as long as the mother and fetus are not moving excessively, the fetus is not too small, or the abdomen is not too large. For long-term monitoring, frequent repositioning of the transducer is generally necessary to track the fetal heart rate. To overcome this, most newer transducers have an array of several pairs of transmitting crystals that generate a wider ultrasound beam.

Direct (Internal) Fetal Heart Rate Monitoring

The direct (internal) method requires that the membranes be ruptured and an electrode placed directly on the fetal scalp. If the patient is not in labor, induction must be commenced. The electrode used at present is a spiral in the form of a helix that has a maximum penetration of 2 mm. The electrodes are disposable and are made of stainless steel. The electrode is placed through the cervix and twisted to imbed in the fetal scalp.

The FHR recorder uses information provided in the electrocardiograph of the infant's heart to quantify the heart rate. Instantaneous beat-to-beat heart rate variations of less than 0.5 beats per minute are detectable using electronic cardiotachometers. Most direct FHR tracings are reliable and accurate.

The FHR can also be followed by auscultation (AUS), that is, by listening with a stethoscope placed against the woman's abdomen or by using a hand-held Doppler device that magnifies the fetal heart tones so that they are audible. These methods require personal attendance to the patient and counting by the observer. They obviously do not create a recording of the FHR and are not continuous. It would certainly appear that continuous EFM is a much more accurate and advanced technology.

Monitoring Uterine Activity

Two main procedures for continuous uterine contraction monitoring are commonly used: external monitoring by tocodynamometer and intrauterine pressure measurements by fluid strain gauge catheterization.

The tocodynamometer is a transducer for the automatic palpation of uterine activity. This is essentially a strain gauge transducer (a round disk with a moveable button that responds to hardening of the uterine wall), held in place over the uterine fundus by an elastic belt. With uterine contractions, the relative pressure against the transducer changes, sending an electrical signal that is recorded on a chart. This technique allows continuous monitoring of the frequency, duration, and relative intensity of the contractions. However, as with palpation, neither the actual intrauterine pressure nor the baseline uterine tone can be determined with current external tocodynamometers.

The correct placement of the tocodynamometer is of critical importance and requires periodic adjustment. When the uterus contracts, the abdominal wall becomes tense and pushes against the transducer. Other motions may exert similar pressure against the transducer. For example, maternal and fetal movements and respirations will also send signals that produce artifactual recordings. Furthermore, if the attachment loosens, signals are inappropriately recorded by the tocodynamometer.

A fluid-filled catheter is used for intrauterine pressure measurements. The catheter is introduced through the cervix, with its distal end immersed in the amniotic fluid and its proximal end immersed in the transducer. The pressure of the amniotic fluid can then be recorded. Pressure readings are accurate only if there is a continuous flow of fluid from the intraamniotic area to the transducer.

This method of intrauterine pressure measurement provides relatively accurate information about the intensity, frequency, and duration of the uterine contractions and about the resting tone between uterine contractions on a continuous basis.

Interpreting Fetal Heart Rates

The reading of the fetal heart rate (FHR) thus depends on a continuous recording of uterine contraction and the FHR on graph paper. Three aspects of the FHR are analyzed: the baseline rate; the periodic fluctuations of the heart rate (accelerations or decelerations), especially as related to uterine contractions; and the beat-to-beat variability, that is, the difference in the heart rate between any two beats.

The patterns are then judged to be reassuring, nonreassuring, or ominous. Reassuring FHR patterns correlate well with excellent fetal status; 99% of infants will not be acidotic. Nonreassuring patterns present a gray area to judgment; the pattern may indicate some fetal problems but usually not. Ominous patterns present such a significant potential for fetal hypoxia and acidosis that intervention or further assessment is essential. Ominous patterns are much less precise in the diagnosis and prediction of actual distress than are reassuring patterns, since only 30% to 40% of infants with ominous tracings will experience hypoxia.

Fetal Blood Sampling

Any discussion of EFM must also include fetal scalp blood sampling (FSBS). Cells require oxygen for function and can only obtain energy for a short time anaerobically. The lack of oxygen leads to a buildup of acids that lower body pH. The combination of decreased oxygen and buildup of acids leads to potential damage to cells and death. Normal pH values vary from 7.35 to 7.25 in normal fetuses. It appears that it takes a pH value in the range of 7.0 or less to cause cell damage.

By placing a plastic cone through the vagina against the fetal head, a puncture can be made and a sample of blood drawn and analyzed for pH. Ranges of 7.25 to 7.20 are considered preacidotic and below 7.20 acidotic, although until the pH is much lower, no evidence of damage occurs. This procedure is thought to be a necessary adjunct to EFM to reduce the overdiagnosis of fetal distress. The technique is difficult, awkward, uncomfortable for women, and technically difficult even with considerable experience.

Efficacy of EFM

Before considering opportunities for improving perinatal outcomes by changing intrapartum management, we must examine the numbers of infants who might be helped. In other words, we must first consider the magnitude of benefit that might result from an optimal use of EFM technology. A number of researchers have suggested that the use of EFM would potentially reduce intrapartum deaths or stillbirths, mental retardation, and cerebral palsy. What is the evidence?

In the United States Collaborative Perinatal Study the total incidence of intrapartum fetal deaths was 4 per 1,000 live births; for term-sized fetuses weighing more than 2,500 grams, the incidence was 1.5 per 1,000.[6] Prematurity has been identified as a significant factor, since 62% of intrapartum deaths occurred in infants weighing less than 2,500 grams. This group, however, represents only 8.2% of all births.[7]

Central nervous system disorders in the form of cerebral palsy and mental retardation have been attributed to perinatal hypoxia. The rates of cerebral palsy are 2.5 per 1,000 in school-aged children, a fairly consistent finding in western industrialized countries. Low birth weight, growth retardation, and various intrapartum events contribute significantly to cerebral palsy, but hypoxia appears to be an independent contributing factor. In the Collaborative Perinatal Study a low birth weight infant (less than 2,500 grams) had a fourfold increased risk of cerebral palsy, and if that infant also had a low 5-minute Apgar score, a sixfold increased risk. It has been estimated that 20% to 40% of cerebral palsy is the result of intrapartum hypoxia.[8]

In the mid-1970s some obstetrical authorities suggested that 50% of mental retardation could be prevented by the use of EFM.[9] Actual surveys of severe mental retardation (IQs of less than 50, representing a biological insult to the brain) are 3 to 4 per 1,000 children. Some of these data are presented in Table 1.

Perinatal events, of which intrapartum hypoxia is only one, cause only approximately 10% of the total cases of severe mental retardation. Some of the other causes are shown in Table 2.

It appears, especially in full-term infants, that even the most severely asphyxiated infants develop normally. About 90% of black and 95% of white

TABLE 1: SELECTED ESTIMATES OF THE PREVALENCE OF SEVERE AND MILD
MENTAL RETARDATION PER 1,000 POPULATION OF A GIVEN AGE

Location	Year of Publication	Age Group	Rate/1,000: Severe	Rate/1,000: Mild
Oregon U.S.	1962	12-14	3.3	30.3
Aberdeen Scotland	1970	8-10	3.7	23.7
Onondaga New York	1955	5-7	3.6	-
Middlesex England	1962	10-14	3.6	-
Quebec Canada	1973	10	3.8	-
Netherlands	1976	19	3.7	31.0
Isle of Wight England	1970	9-14	-	25.3

From: Antenatal Diagnosis, Report of a Consensus Conference,
        National Institute of Child Health and Human Development,
        NIH, Bethesda, Maryland, U.S. Dept. of HEW, NIH Publication
        No. 80-1973, 1979.

TABLE 2: THE ESTIMATED CURRENT DISTRIBUTION (%) OF SELECTED CAUSES
OF SEVERE MENTAL RETARDATION IN DEVELOPED COUNTRIES

Cause	Distribution Reported	Inferred
1. Chromosomal anomaly	36	36
2. Congenital malformation syndromes with recurrence risks	20	27
3. Genetic metabolic errors	7	8
4. Prenatal	8	8
5. Perinatal causes: birth, trauma, hypoxia, hyperbilirubinemia, hypoglycemia, intracranial hemorrhage	8	9
6. Infections:		
prenatal	2	4
perinatal	2	5
postnatal	2	3

From: *Antenatal Diagnosis*, Report of a Consensus Conference, National Institute of Child Health and Human Development, NIH, Bethesda, Maryland, U.S. Dept. of HEW, NIH Publication No. 80-1973, 1979.

surviving children in the Collaborative Perinatal Study who had 5-minute Apgar scores of 3 or less were found to be of normal intelligence several years later.[10]

The National Institute of Child Health and Human Development task force, in evaluating the available data, estimated that the maximum number of cases of cerebral palsy and severe mental retardation potentially preventable through the universal use of EFM to be 1 per 1,000 live births in all categories of risk. Thus the numbers at risk for intrapartum death and for hypoxial brain damage are very low and especially so in low-risk, full-term pregnancies. Indeed, Dr. Mark Thompson, in a recent proposal,[11] calculated that to do a study of the difference in perinatal death rates between full-term, low-risk monitored and unmonitored patients would require the analysis of 180,000 patients in each group. The very size of the required groups casts doubt on the need for universal use of EFM, since obviously very low incidence problems are involved. Furthermore, the possible adverse effects resulting from the use of EFM would also warrant careful consideration.

Review of EFM Studies

The questions that can be asked about EFM are the following: (1) How does it affect perinatal mortality? (2) How does it affect perinatal morbidity, including any immediate outcome and long-term neurological function? (3) How does it affect maternal morbidity, and especially cesarean section rates? In attempting to answer these questions, we can review the data presently available from retrospective studies, analytical studies, and randomized controlled trials.

In the following discussion, the term "retrospective trials" will refer to studies in which data from different time periods (pre-EFM and post-EFM) were compared. The "analytical studies" are those in which part of an obstetrical service used EFM while the rest of the service did not, and the outcome of each of these two "treatments" was compared. "Randomized controlled trials" are prospective studies in which patients are randomly assigned to treatment groups (EFM or auscultation) at the same time, in one setting, cared for by the same personnel, and outcomes compared.

Perinatal mortality decreased from 32.5 in 1950 to 20.1 in 1973 to 11.3 in 1979. Some authors have attributed a large proportion of this decline to the introduction of EFM. Although it is difficult to identify the fraction of contribution of any new strategy to an outcome that is influenced by so many different factors, we can at least think about the efficacy of a given technique and the evidence of its success.

Perinatal mortality is subject to a variety of influences, making it difficult to single out any one factor as causal. For example, during the period that EFM was being introduced, perinatal mortality was being influenced by the use of contraceptives, an increase in abortion, better nutrition, patient education, better prenatal and obstetrical care, and genetic counseling. Increased attention during labor and delivery may very easily reduce perinatal mortality. Obstetrical practice itself was changing with the use of ultrasound, amniocentesis, an increased use of cesarean section, including the decreased utilization of traumatic delivery techniques such as midforceps. Finally, the neonatal period is the most critical period with respect to the occurrence of mortality. Perhaps it is the improved neonatal care provided by the neonatologist that has been most responsible for reducing neonatal death.

EFM Studies of Intrapartum Fetal Death Rates

Intrapartum fetal death (IFD) is defined as the death during labor of a fetus who has been positively identified by the presence of fetal heart rate as alive at the start of labor. Almost all of the retrospective and analytical studies show a significant decrease in IFD following the use of EFM. The four major retrospective studies show that EFM is followed by 2.5 fewer deaths per 1,000 live births than auscultation.[8] In other words, they all reach the conclusion that fetal lives were saved during labor.

In the four randomized controlled trials,[12-15] there were 2,032 subjects of whom 899 were followed by auscultation and 1,133 by EFM. In Renou's study, one intrapartum death occurred in the auscultated group. It should be noted that in the general literature, 60% of intrapartum deaths occur among premature infants. Term pregnancy rates are about 1.5 per 1,000. With respect to term pregnancy, even among "high-risk" mothers, it would be necessary to study 20,000 cases in order to show differences in intrapartum fetal death rates. Thus it is not surprising that with their smaller sample sizes, none of the four randomized controlled trials shows any effect of EFM on the incidence of intrapartum fetal deaths.

In summary, the randomized controlled trials reveal no significant differences in intrapartum fetal death but are too small in size to permit any inferences. The large retrospective and analytical studies collectively observed more than 70,000 cases. Although less rigorous in design than controlled trials, their size must be respected. They reveal significant differences in outcome between EFM and non-EFM groups. It is our belief that the strongest justification for electronic fetal monitoring comes from the reductions in intrapartum fetal death rates, as learned from the retrospective and analytical studies.

The four randomized controlled trials (Table 3) showed no reduction in perinatal mortality. There were 2 deaths among 899 auscultated patients and 4 deaths among the 1,133 mothers who were electronically monitored.

Some comments must be made concerning low birth weight infants. Neutra and co-workers performed a multivariate analysis of data characterizing 16,529 live-born infants delivered at Beth Israel Hospital in Boston over a 7-year period.[16] They estimated the neonatal death rates and found that the failure to use EFM increased the risk of neonatal death 1.7 times. However, the benefit occurred only among the high risk and low birth weight infants. Among the 12,055 lowest risk patients, the neonatal death rates were lower in the auscultated group (0.5 per 1,000) than in the EFM groups (1.1 per 1,000). Other analytical studies[17,18] have suggested significant benefits for EFM to the grossly premature infant, but no controlled trials have been done in this birth weight range.

Perinatal Mortality

Evaluation of neonatal death rates is complicated by the many changes that have occurred in neonatal intensive care. The retrospective studies did not show a beneficial effect on neonatal death rates following the use of EFM.

TABLE 3: CAUSE AND DISTRIBUTION OF SIX PERINATAL DEATHS (EXCLUDING MAJOR CONGENITAL ABNORMALITIES) AMONG 2,032 PATIENTS IN RCT's BY STUDY CENTER AND STUDY GROUP

	Intermittent Auscultation	Continuous Electronic Monitoring	Continuous Electronic Monitoring + Biochemical Assessment
Denver (1973-1975)	(N=241) ---	(N=242) Meconium aspiration	0 ---
Melbourne (1974-1975)	(N=175) Intrapartum asphyxia	0 ---	(N=175) Pulmonary Haemorrhage
Denver (1975-1977)	(N=232) ---	(N=233) Intracranial Haemorrhage	(N=230) Septicaemia
Sheffield (1976-1977)	(N=251) Meconium aspiration	0 ---	(N=253) ---

From: Chalmers, I. Randomized, controlled trials of intrapartum fetal monitoring, 6th European Congress of Perinatal Medicine, Vienna, Austria, 1978, Georg Thieme Verlag, Stuttgart.

Neonatal Morbidity

Unlike perinatal mortality, some forms of perinatal morbidity occur frequently enough to permit comparisons of exposed and unexposed groups in randomized controlled trials. Information as to 1- and 5-minute Apgar scores, biochemical status of the infant at birth (as measured by cord pH, PO_2 and PCO_2) and immediate neonatal neurological status are available for comparison in Table 4.

All four randomized controlled trials included a comparison of low 1- and 5-minute Apgar scores; there were no significant differences in scores between EFM and auscultated groups. The two Denver randomized controlled trials were the only studies with complete cord blood gas measurements.

In 1,178 patients studied in two separate trials, there were absolutely no differences in any fetal blood gas measurements between the EFM and the auscultated groups. Renou[15] did find some differences, but only sampled

84 out of 350 patients and only between 9:00 A.M. and 5:00 P.M., when the laboratory was open. Kelso,[14] in the British study, states that no differences were found but does not provide these data. In 1980, Wood and colleagues[19] conducted a second controlled trial in a low-risk obstetrical population, once more showing no differences in perinatal outcome.

Only one of the studies followed-up the infants beyond the time of their birth. In the second Denver trial, infants were examined at 9 months to see whether differences in health and neurological status, not visible at birth, were apparent later. Pediatric, motor, and mental examinations along with

TABLE 4: COMPARISON OF PERINATAL MORTALITY AND MORBIDITY BETWEEN MATCHED GROUPS OF WOMEN MONITORED ELECTRONICALLY AND BY AUSCULTATION IN THE FOUR RANDOMIZED CONTROLLED TRIALS (RCT's)

	Haverkamp N=483	Renou N=350	Haverkamp N=695	Kelso N=504
Perinatal mortality in EFM vs auscultated	no difference	no difference	no difference	no difference
Apgar score EFM vs auscultated	no difference	no difference	no difference	no difference
Cord blood pH in EFM vs auscultated	no difference	claimed better in EFM*	no difference	no difference
Neonatal neurologic abnormalities EFM vs auscultated	no difference	0 in EFM 4 in auscultated**	no difference	no difference
Neurologic abnormalities in long-term follow-up	no difference	no follow-up published	no difference	no follow-up

* Cord blood pH measurements were done among auscultated newborn infants only if they were born during the 9:00 A.M. to 5:00 P.M. hours that the hospital laboratory was open.

** There were 5 difficult forceps extractions among the auscultated infants, and none among the electronically monitored infants. The four newborns with neonatal convulsions were among the five infants delivered with midforceps.

From: Banta, D., Thacker, S. Electronic fetal monitoring: is it of benefit, Birth Fam J 6: 237-249, 1979.

health history results were compared, and no differences were found between the EFM and auscultated groups.

Neurological Effects

No neurological data are available from the analytical or retrospective studies. Neonatal neurological examination was done in each of the four controlled trials, and differences between auscultated and EFM groups were found only in Renou's study. Four large-size term infants in the auscultated group exhibited significant neurological damage, but since all four had experienced traumatic second stages during labor and were delivered with mid-forceps, it would appear that trauma was a causal factor, not the fetal surveillance. In the second Haverkamp trial a pediatrician, who did not know the study group origins of the infants, performed the neonatal assessments at the time of birth. No differences in neurological problems between EFM and non-EFM groups of infants were found, nor was there an apparent need for neonatal intensive care. Infants were examined at 9 months, and their Bayley and Milani-Comparetti test scores were not significantly different. These tests are commonly used measures of mental and motor functions.

The only study correlating abnormal FHR patterns with neurological outcome was conducted by Painter and co-workers,[20] who found that ominous fetal heart rate patterns predicted abnormal neurological performances more accurately than did Apgar scores. However, in an analysis of the prospective data in the second Denver trial, no correlation could be found between ominous FHR patterns and abnormal neurological outcomes unless there were other contributing factors. Many times EFM identifies infants who are already damaged by congenital or prepartum factors. Indeed, EFM may lead to the rescue of infants seriously ill with cerebral palsy or anomalies such as trisomy 18, which result in prolonged hospitalizations, ending in inevitable early death or lifetime disabilities.

As was mentioned earlier, serious questions have been raised about both the assumption that intrapartum anoxia is a cause of motor and intellectual disability and that EFM, by detecting anoxia earlier, can thereby prevent such disability. Although Adamsons and Myers[21] have demonstrated a clear association between severe, prolonged late decelerations and reduced fetal blood oxygen, they have also shown that the healthy term monkey can tolerate such a reduction for many hours without any clinical or morphological sequelae. Primate research shows that the threshold of severity of asphyxia required to produce brain injury is so close to that required to produce fetal death that asphyxia is nearly always followed by complete recovery or the death of the fetus. This "all-or-nothing" effect is suggested by several authors[22-24] and confirmed both by primate and human infant studies. When term infants who had experienced intrapartum hypoxia were compared with others who did not, no differences in physical or mental scores at 4 years of age were found.[25]

EFM and the Cesarean Section Rate

During the period of introduction and adaptation of EFM, the cesarean section rate has increased more than threefold, from 5% in 1970 to 16.5% in 1980.[26] It is interesting that some of the same authorities who claim EFM has decreased the perinatal mortality during this time also say that EFM is not related to the increased cesarean section rate.[27,28] However, the analytical studies (comparing EFM and auscultation at the same time) and the retrospective studies (comparing several different years) show dramatic increases in cesarean section rates (Tables 5 to 7).

Only one retrospective study of fetal monitoring, a British study by

TABLE 5: ANALYTIC STUDIES: COMPARISON OF CESAREAN SECTION RATES AMONG WOMEN MONITORED BY AUSCULTATION AND THOSE MONITORED BY ELECTRONIC FETAL MONITORS (EFM)*

Studies	% Auscultated	% EFM
Paul, et al (1977)	7	9.5
Tutera and Newman (1975)	5	10
Kelly and Kulkarni (1973)	8	18
Gassner and Ledger (1976)	7	15
Hill (1972)	6	15
Amato (1977)	6	9

* In some of these studies women monitored by EFM are at greater risk than those monitored by auscultation. Therefore, a higher Cesarean rate may partly reflect Cesareans indicated for reasons other than fetal monitoring patterns.

From: Banta, D., Thacker, S. Electronic fetal monitoring: is it of benefit, Birth Fam J 6: 237-249, 1979.

Beard,[27] showed a decrease in cesarean section rates, and the randomized controlled trials all showed significant increases in the cesarean section rates.

Increased rates occurred among both high- and low-risk populations. Haverkamp's Denver studies showed cesarean section rates of 6% for auscultated and 18% for EFM groups. For 1,000 term high-risk women, this implies that 120 more cesarean sections would occur if EFM were used. An increased rate of cesarean section occurred for both the diagnosis of fetal distress and dystocia. The rate for fetal distress was 1% among auscultated mothers compared with 6% among EFM mothers. Cesarean sections occurred among 5% of the auscultated mothers but were doubled to 10% among EFM mothers.

In national statistics, as mentioned earlier, cesarean section rates have more than tripled between 1970 and 1980.[26] These statistics seem to mirror an identical trend seen in the prospective trials of the increasing diagnosis of fetal distress and dystocia with EFM. In the case of primary cesarean sec-

TABLE 6: RETROSPECTIVE STUDIES: COMPARISON OF CESAREAN
SECTION RATES AMONG WOMEN BEFORE AND AFTER THE
INTRODUCTION OF ELECTRONIC FETAL MONITORS (EFM)*

	% Before EFM	% After EFM
Lee and Baggish (1976)	7	10
Heldfond et al. (1976)	5	13
Koh et al. (1975)	6	12.5
Shenker et al. (1975)	3	6.5
Gabert & Stenchever (1973)	3.5	9
Fleet et al. (1976)	4	12.5
Beard et al. (1977)	9	6

* Monitoring was not the only factor to change during the
period of 1968-1977. More Cesareans were done for breech
presentation, premature delivery and other indications.

From: Banta, H.D., Thacker, S.B. Assessing the costs and
benefits of electronic fetal monitoring, Ob/Gyn Surv.
35:627-42, 1979.

The Williams & Wilkins Company, Baltimore.

TABLE 7: COMPARISON OF CESAREAN SECTION RATES BETWEEN
MATCHED GROUPS OF WOMEN MONITORED ELECTRONICALLY
AND BY AUSCULTATION IN THE FOUR RANDOMIZED
CONTROLLED TRIALS

	%	%	%
	AUS	EFM	EFM/FBS SAMPLING
Haverkamp (N=483)	7	17	-
Renou (N=350)	14	-	22
Haverkamp (N=695)	6	18	12
Kelso (N=504)	4	9	-

tion between 1970 and 1978, 40% of the rise is attributable to the diagnosis and response to dystocia, whereas 28% of the cesarean sections are for "other fetal" problems including fetal distress (Table 8).

As can be seen in Table 8, breech births contribute significantly to increased cesareans, and the total cesarean section rate would appear to be strongly influenced by the traditional dictum, "Once a section always a section." In other words, there would appear to be a multiplier effect, since once a cesarean section is done, all subsequent pregnancies will be delivered by repeat surgery. In 1978, 99% of women who had a cesarean section were delivered by a repeat procedure. Whether or not this is necessary is another question.

There are several studies of low-profile care given to low-risk women in labor without using EFM. Goodlin[23] published the results of a study of 500 consecutive patients cared for in a tertiary hospital by nurse-midwives, without EFM. The cesarean section rate was 2.8%. Each patient was matched against the next normal low-risk patient, cared for by usual hospital procedures, including EFM, and the primary cesarean section rate rose to 9.2%. Lehrfeld[29] noted that patients (including 48% primigravidas) who were observed without EFM, had a cesarean section rate of 3.4%, whereas at the same time in Boston in a high-technology hospital employing EFM universally, 45% of primigravidas had cesarean sections.

There seem to be two principal reasons why fetal monitoring engenders increased cesarean sections: (1) an increase in the diagnosis of fetal distress, and (2) an increased diagnosis of dystocia. The fetal monitor cannot always

TABLE 8: CONTRIBUTION TO RISE IN CESAREAN DELIVERY RATES
FROM 1970 TO 1978 OF CHANGES IN CESAREAN DELIVERY
RATES AND PERCENT DELIVERIES WITH COMPLICATIONS,
EXCLUSIVE OF PREVIOUS CESAREAN DELIVERY

Complication	Contribution to Rise Total
No mention	0.0
Lacerations	1.5
Dystocia (1)	40.0
Breech	21.5
Persistent occiput posterior	1.5
Other malpresentations	3.0
Other "maternal" (2)	1.6
Other "fetal" (3)	27.7
Other fetal - both years (4)	(10.8)
Other unspecified	3.1
All of the above	100.0

(1) Fetopelvic disproportion, abnormal pelvis, prolonged labor.
(2) Antepartum hemorrhage, prior gynecological surgery.
(3) Premature ROM, premature labor, multiple, prolonged ROM, prolonged pregnancy, fetal distress.
(4) Premature ROM, premature labor

From: Draft Report of the Task Force on Cesarean Childbirth, U.S. Dept. of HHS, PHS, NIH, 1980, p. 127.

distinguish the difference between stress and distress of the fetus. Only 30% to 40% of the time, with ominous fetal heart rate patterns, are the infants actually acidotic. There is a tendency to overcall fetal distress, based on a fetal heart rate pattern, which on review, is not ominous at all. Finally, the fetal heart rate monitor, continually present at the bedside, along with the interaction between the patient, nurse, partner, and physician may induce stresses that contribute to fetal distress in the infant.

Monitor-associated dystocia appears to be as significant a contributor to cesarean sections as fetal distress. The reasons for the increased diagnosis of dystocia with EFM might well be the following:

1. EFM restricts activity. In particular, the external monitor forces a woman to lie on her back. If she moves very much, the fetal heart rate sign is lost.

2. Overly strict criteria are used for what is termed "failure to progress" with a monitor in place. If external monitors are used, they tend to make contractions appear more effective (on the graph paper) than they may actually be. This may be more true when a tocodynamometer is tightly attached.

Summary

In summary, it can be said that there are both positive and negative aspects in the use of EFM. The positive aspects can be described as follows:

1. EFM allows physicians and nurses experienced in its use instantaneously to assess fetal status during labor.
2. EFM permits the detection of subtle changes in infant asphyxia that auscultation may miss. For instance, it can detect late decelerations and a lack of beat-to-beat variability.
3. Reassuring FHR patterns correlate with good infant outcomes (99%).
4. Ominous FHR patterns correlate with acidosis and asphyxia (30%).
5. EFM heightens the attention to the fetus.

The negative aspects can be described as follows:

1. EFM increases cesarean sections, some unnecessary, for reasons of fetal distress and dystocia.
2. EFM patterns are not easy to read:
   a. Normal or reassuring FHR patterns are sometimes miscalled ominous.
   b. Subtle ominous patterns can be missed.
3. Ominous FHR patterns overcall fetal distress, for example, as with late decelerations where only 30% of infants may be acidotic, whereas 70% are normal.
4. Monitors restrict patient movement. EFM, especially external monitors, tends to force patients to remain flat on their backs in labor.
5. Monitors seem to, but should not, replace nurses as caregivers in labor.
6. The monitor becomes the focus for partners, nurses, and physicians rather than the woman in labor.
7. The monitor medicalizes labor and appears to interfere with freedom, relaxation, and motion, producing what some have called negative biofeedback or anxiety that tends to interrupt labor.

In conclusion, almost all the retrospective and analytical studies show a dramatic rise in the cesarean section rate with the use of EFM, as do all of the randomized trials. This finding is reflected in national statistics in the United States on the increase in cesarean section rates. Under usual practice today, the use of EFM appears to at least double the rate of cesarean section in otherwise uncomplicated pregnancies—a matter of serious concern to society and to obstetrics in the 1980s.

Recommendations

Obviously there are tensions and concerns with respect to the use of EFM, and many nurses and physicians are so accustomed to its use on all patients that they are uncomfortable without it. Based on our own experiences with EFM, the findings of the controlled trials, and the recognition of the negative aspects of EFM, the following recommendations can be made for its selective use:

1. The use of continuous EFM should be selectively applied to high-risk patients.
2. For low-risk term patients, a 10-minute monitoring strip should be run on women in labor upon admission. EFM detects 1 to 2 per 1,000 fetuses with problems at the time of admission.
3. With reassuring FHR patterns, the monitor may be removed and fetal status followed at 15- to 30-minute intervals by
   a. auscultation
   b. Doppler ultrasound
   c. external FHR monitor
4. After complete dilatation, the FHR should be determined every 5 minutes in the second stage of labor.
5. Artificial rupture of the membranes and internal EFM should be used only for specific indications of risk.
6. All obstetrical personnel should periodically review FHR patterns and tracings to develop and/or maintain their skills.
7. Fetal blood scalp sampling should be used in conjunction with EFM to avoid false positive diagnoses of fetal distress and, thereby, unnecessary cesarean sections.

REFERENCES

1. Banta HD, Thacker SB. Assessing the costs and benefits of electronic fetal monitoring. *Ob/Gyn Surv* 35:627–642, 1979.

2. Hearings before the Subcommittee on Health and Scientific Research of the Committee on Human Resources, United States Senate. *Obstetrical Practices in the United States, 1978,* Washington, DC, US Government Printing Office.

3. Russell LB. *Technology in hospitals: Medical advances and their diffusion.* Washington, DC, The Brookings Institution, 1979.

4. Altman SH, and Blendon R (eds). *Medical technology: The culprit behind health care costs?* Proceedings of 1977 Sun Valley Forum on National Health, 1979.

5. *Health United States, 1980,* US Department of Health and Human Services, Public Health Service, Office of Health Research, Statistics and Technology, pp 29–33, 1980.

6. Lilien A. Term intrapartum fetal death rates. *Am J Obstet Gynecol* 107:595–603, 1970.

7. Chase HC. Perinatal mortality: Overview and current trends. *Clin Perinatol* 1:3–17, 1974.

8. *Antenatal diagnosis,* Report of a Consensus Conference, National Institute of Child Health and Human Development, NIH, Bethesda, MD, US Department of Health, Education, and Welfare, Publication No.79-1973, 1979.

9. Quilligan EJ, Paul RH. Fetal monitoring, is it worth it? *Obstet Gynecol* 45:96–100, 1975.

10. Broman S: Perinatal anoxia and cognitive development in early childhood. In Field T, Sostek AM, Goldberg S, et al (eds). *Infants born at risk*, Englewood Cliffs, NJ, Spectrum Books, 1978.

11. Thompson M, Cohen AB. *Uncertainty concerning electronic fetal monitoring*, working draft, April, 1980.

12. Haverkamp AD, Orleans M, Langendoerfer S, et al. A controlled trial of the differential effects of intrapartum fetal monitoring. *Am J Obstet Gynecol* 134:399–408, 1979.

13. Haverkamp AD, Thompson HE, McFee JG, et al. The evaluation of continuous fetal heart rate monitoring in high-risk pregnancy. *Am J Obstet Gynecol* 125:310–320, 1976.

14. Kelso AM, Parsons RJ, Lawrence GT, et al. An assessment of continuous fetal heart rate monitoring in labor. *Am J Obstet Gynecol* 131:526–532, 1978.

15. Renou R, Chang A, Anderson I, et al. Controlled trial of fetal intensive care. *Am J Obstet Gynecol* 126:470–476, 1976.

16. Neutra R, Fienberg SE, Greenland S. The effect of fetal monitoring on neonatal death rates. *N Engl J Med* 299:324–326, 1978.

17. Hobel CJ, Hyvarinem OW. Abnormal fetal heart rate patterns and fetal acid base balance in low birth weight infants in relation to respiratory distress syndrome. *Obstet Gynecol* 39:83, 1972.

18. Martin CB, Siassi B, and Hon EH. Fetal heart rate patterns and neonatal death in low birthweight infants. *Obstet Gynecol* 44:150–153, 1974.

19. Wood C, Renou P, Oats J, et al. A controlled trial of fetal heart rate monitoring in a low-risk obstetric population. *Am J Obstet Gynecol* 141:527–534, 1981.

20. Painter MJ, Depp R, and O'Donoghue PD. Fetal heart rate patterns and development in the first year of life. *Am J Obstet Gynecol* 132:271–277, 1978.

21. Adamsons K, Myers RE. Late decelerations and brain tolerance of the fetal monkey to intrapartum asphyxia. *Am J Obstet Gynecol* 128:893–900, 1977.

22. Davies P, Stewart A. Low birth-weight infants: Neurological sequelae. *Br Med Bull* 31:85–91, 1975.

23. Goodlin RC, Haesslein HC. When is it fetal distress? *Am J Obstet Gynecol* 128:440–447, 1977.

24. Low J, Galbraith R, Muir D, et al. Intrapartum fetal asphyxia: Preliminary report in regard to long-term morbidity. *Am J Obstet Gynecol* 130:525–533, 1978.

25. Niswander K, Gordon M, Drage J. The effect of intrauterine hypoxia in the child surviving to four years. *Am J Obstet Gynecol* 121:892–899, 1975.

26. Placek PJ, Taffel SM. One-sixth of 1980 U.S. births by caesarean section. *Public Health Rep* 97:183, Mar–Apr, 1982.

27. Beard RW, Edington PT, Sibanda J. The effects of routine intrapartum monitoring on clinical practice. *Contrib Gynecol Obstet* 3:14–21, 1977.

28. Paul RH, Huey JR, Yeay CF. Clinical fetal monitoring, its effect on cesarean section rate and perinatal mortality: Five year trends. *Postgrad Med* 61:160–166, 1977.

29. Lehrfeld J. Presentation at District 8 Meeting of The American College Obstetricians and Gynecologists, Colorado Springs, Oct, 1980.

SUBMITTED: JANUARY, 1982
REVISED & ACCEPTED: AUGUST, 1982

OBSTETRICAL ANALGESIA AND ANESTHESIA

Paul L. Doering

Over 130 years have passed since chloroform and ether were first used in childbirth in the quest for the "painless delivery."[1] Since then, numerous other anesthetic and analgesic agents have become available. Some of these have proved to have a favorable effect on the outcome of labor, whereas others have produced harmful consequences. Today, there is a host of obstetrical medications, including anesthetics, analgesics, sedatives, antinauseants, preanesthetic agents, and a variety of adjunctive agents.

Although the notion of decreased pain and anxiety during labor and delivery is initially appealing, relief must not be accomplished at the the expense of maternal and fetal well-being. Yet it is now known that some drugs once considered "routine" or "standard" for the woman in labor are, in fact, the direct cause of morbidity and mortality for both the mother and child. Thus drugs can be viewed as a two-edged sword: On the one side they can ease the pain of childbirth, resulting in a more rapid, less anxiety-filled delivery, whereas on the other they can produce serious injury. Clearly, drugs should be used only when their expected benefits justify the risks that accompany any pharmacological intervention.

But how can the patient participate in this benefit-to-risk determination? Should not this determination be left to the physician? Perhaps that was the prevailing attitude in the past, but it is not the case in the 1980s. The patient must have input into the decision-making process, since it is ultimately her body and that of her baby which will be affected. This chapter is intended to provide the information to allow women and their labor partners to be better decision makers about the obstetrical use of drugs.

Placental Transport of Drugs

The placenta is a specialized organ that functions as the point of junction between the mother and her developing fetus. Although fetal and maternal blood ordinarily do not physically mix, this organ is the site of transport of nutrients, oxygen, and essential hormones and other constituents from the mother to the infant. Likewise, the placenta transports fetal carbon dioxide and other metabolic waste products from the baby's blood into the mother's circulation for ultimate elimination. Structurally, the placenta is an organized network of capillaries with fetal attachment and is bathed by maternal blood. At the cellular level, its transport function is accomplished in a manner similar to that of other biological membranes.

In the past the placental unit was often referred to as the "placental barrier." Modern science has confirmed, however, that the organ is more accurately described as a "selective sieve." In fact, most drugs and other chemicals readily cross the placenta and enter the fetal circulation. It is now recognized that drugs excluded by the placenta are the exceptions and not the rule.[2]

Most substances cross the placenta by a process of passive diffusion whereby a substance which is at a higher concentration in one compartment (e.g., maternal blood) will move from that compartment to one of lower concentration (e.g., fetal blood) when separated by biological membranes. With few exceptions, all endogenous and exogenous chemicals cross the placenta to some degree by passive diffusion.

The extent and ease with which drugs traverse the placenta depends on several characteristics of the compound in question. Molecular size, electrical charge, concentration gradient, lipid solubility of the drug, degree of binding to blood proteins, and the acid/base status of the mother and fetus can all influence the amount of a drug that ends up in the fetal environment. Most drugs are of relatively small molecular size so that they can pass through "pores" in the placenta. Similarly, the other attributes of most drugs favor transport rather than exclusion of the agent.

Keeping this in mind, one needs to focus one's attention on the consequences after the drug has entered the child's plasma. On the one hand, it is not always undesirable for a drug to get into fetal circulation. For example, penicillin administered to a pregnant woman with syphilis readily crosses the placenta and is found in high concentrations in fetal blood. This is considered beneficial, since the baby is receiving treatment concurrent with the mother. Likewise, a condition known as idiopathic fetal tachycardia is a problem that may be treated by administering digoxin to the mother, since digoxin readily passes the placenta and produces equal maternal and fetal serum concentrations.[3] On the other hand, some drugs can enter the fetal circulation and persist in the infant's body even after delivery. Diazepam (Valium), for example, is eliminated slowly from the infant's body and may cause drowsiness and lethargy for several days after delivery.[4] Thus many drugs cross the placenta, but not all have adverse consequences.

Mechanism of Drug Effects on the Fetus

There are several basic mechanisms by which drugs used during pregnancy, labor, and delivery can cause adverse effects.

Physical malformations. Drugs have their most profound effects when given during the first trimester of pregnancy. This is the period when embryological differentiation of the organ systems is occurring, and insult by certain chemicals and drugs (e.g., thalidomide) can interrupt this process, causing physical malformations in the fetus. There is a wide variation in the reported frequency of drug-induced physical malformations. The usual estimate is that 1% to 3% of the newborn population has some deviation from normal morphology from all causes and that drugs and environmental chemicals account for an estimated 2% to 3% of these.[5]

Indeed, the true incidence is difficult if not impossible to determine, given the limitations of research with pregnant women and the logistical problems in monitoring large numbers of women to detect adverse effects. Drugs administered during labor and delivery are usually not responsible for physical malformations, since by this time the fetus has passed the stage where organ development occurs.

Pharmacological effects. Drugs given to the mother during labor can be expected to be in the fetal circulation at the time the baby is born. The fetus therefore is likely to respond to the medication in the same fashion as the mother. For example, narcotics such as morphine or its derivatives are well known to depress the depth as well as rate of respirations in adults who are given relatively large doses.[6] There is no reason to expect these effects to be any less pronounced in the neonate. In fact, there is some evidence that certain drugs actually accumulate in the baby's blood, resulting in an exaggerated or prolonged response.

General anesthetics carry the risk of producing a sleepy baby because, after all, the therapeutic endpoint of treatment for the mother is sleep. It would be desirable if drug effects could be isolated to the mother but as long as the drug crosses into fetal circulation, it has the potential to cause the same effect in the infant as in the mother.

The timing of administration, dosage, and inherent toxicity of the compound all determine how intensely the infant will react to a drug. These factors will be discussed in detail later.

Alterations of maternal physiology. Some drugs may produce harm to the fetus by altering a physiological process necessary to maintain normal fetal well-being. For instance, drugs that alter placental blood flow may endanger the fetus by decreasing delivery of oxygen and nutrients to the fetus. If oxytocin, a hormone used to induce labor, is given in too great a dose or if the woman is overly sensitive to its effects, the uterus will contract and remain contracted.[7] These "tetanic contractions" do not allow the normal periodic uterine relaxation between contractions. Since during the peak of a contraction uterine blood flow is interrupted, the periods of relaxation are necessary to reestablish flow of blood through the placenta and deliver needed oxygen to the fetus. Prolonged oxygen deprivation may result in brain injury to the child.[7]

Drugs that cause a detrimental change in maternal vital functions may also affect the infant. Although local anesthetic drugs used during spinal and epidural anesthesia do not enter the fetal environment to any large degree, they still may adversely affect infant outcome. A side effect of spinal or epidural anesthesia is a decreased blood pressure, in some cases to a dangerously low level. If maternal blood pressure is reduced too excessively, blood flow to the placenta can be compromised. Again, oxygen deliver is impaired, and if intervention is not initiated, a resultant hypoxic injury to the fetus may occur. Effects of epidural and spinal anesthesia will be discussed in detail in a subsequent section.

Differences in fetal drug metabolism. Drugs and other chemicals are recognized by the body as foreign substances and, as such, are handled in a way that facilitates their removal or inactivation. For example, many drugs are converted by the liver into inactive or less toxic chemicals for ultimate excretion from the body. Other drugs are excreted unchanged by the kidney. Almost all drugs are handled in one or both of these manners.

But the capacity of the body to process and eliminate certain drugs may depend on the functional development of the liver and kidneys. Newborns, especially premature infants, have yet to develop maximum ability to metabolize certain drugs. Drug metabolizing function of the liver has not reached full functional capacity until some time after birth, the time period depending on the specific drug and its metabolic pathway.[8] Renal function is also below maximum at birth.[9] Thus drugs handled by the liver and some excreted by the kidneys can be expected to accumulate if drug elimination pathways are operating at less than full efficiency. Diazepam (Valium) is metabolized by the newborn liver more slowly than the adult liver; therefore diazepam persists in neonatal plasma for periods of several days after birth, causing a prolonged lethargy in the baby.[4] Also, one of the metabolic breakdown products of meperidine (Demerol) is removed slowly from the newborn's body and may serve as a residual source for toxicity.[10]

Effects on the progress of labor. Almost all of the drugs used during the course of labor can affect the frequency and intensity of uterine contractions if given inappropriately. Excessively large doses of narcotics given before a good labor has been established can effectively stop labor.[11] The ideal sedative or analgesic agent would have no effect on normal dilatation and effacement patterns.

Developmental effects on the neonate. There is a growing body of evidence that drugs can injure the newborn's central nervous system (CNS) even in the absence of structural or physiological effects. The baby's CNS is not completely developed at birth; in fact, authors estimate that the period of rapid CNS growth continues for at least 18 months after birth.[12] Drugs can interfere with normal maturation of the CNS and can produce abnormalities in the behavioral capacities of the child.

Behavioral effects are usually detected clinically at school age and may therefore escape association with a drug used years earlier. Also, the effects are far more subtle than other effects and, in some cases, may be demonstrable only with very sensitive testing. A variety of developmental measures have been shown to be affected, at least transiently, by drugs used during labor. These include tests of perception, attention, muscular strength, motor coordination, habituation to auditory, visual, and tactile stimuli, and several other measures.[13-15] Neurological-behavioral test scores from the Brazelton, the Scanlon, and the Bayley scales have all reportedly shown effects from obstetrical drugs.[16-18] The overall implications of the behavioral effects of drugs are still being determined.

Factors Affecting a Drug's Toxicity

As pointed out earlier, drugs can manifest toxicity in a variety of ways, but many women can go through labor receiving numerous drugs and give birth to ''normal'' babies. What factors, then, lead drugs to produce toxicity under certain circumstances and spare the fetus under others?

Inherent effects of the drugs. Some drugs are inherently more toxic than others based on the pharmacological effects they produce. As noted, most analgesics, in addition to reducing pain, also have the ability to affect the central nervous system, depressing respiratory, cardiovascular, or muscle-motor function.

Two drugs from the same pharmacological class may differ in their propensity to produce CNS effects, thus forming a basis for perhaps selecting one over the other. However, many drugs (e.g., the opiates) possess essentially the same toxic potential when they are used in equianalgesic doses.[19]. This is true even though some members of the class are more "potent" on a milligram-for-milligram basis.

Dose. Higher doses of obstetrical medications yield correspondingly higher drug levels in the fetal environment. For most drugs there is a good correlation between amount in the blood and the effects seen. Doses of drugs normally used in the nonpregnant woman may produce neonatal CNS depression when given to the laboring woman if there is no downward dosage adjustment.

Arguments against dosage decreases have centered on concern for loss of efficacy. Some clinicians ask, "If you are going to give such a small dose, why give it at all?" Indeed, there is a dose so low that the therapeutic response is lost. Unfortunately, predicting this dose for an individual woman is difficult. It is better to titrate the dosage upward while monitoring for toxicity than to give arbitrarily high doses, which produce toxicity, and wish that a smaller dose had been given.

The therapeutic endpoint for drugs used to treat subjective complaints such as pain, nausea, and anxiety is difficult to assess. When has an acceptable level of pain relief been achieved? Without knowing a patient's tolerance to pain and being unable to gauge the endpoint, it is best to risk having subtherapeutic doses than toxic doses.

Timing of administration. The entry of drugs into fetal circulation and their ultimate removal by metabolism and excretion all follow a defined time course. Ideally, a drug should be given at a time when its intended effects can be realized and yet there is still time for the compound to be eliminated from maternal and fetal blood. Unfortunately, this is difficult, since one cannot predict in advance exactly when birth will occur.

No drug should be given so early in the labor process that it will inhibit normal progress. As a rule of thumb, analgesics, sedatives, antinauseants, and other drugs with depressant properties should not be administered before the cervix is dilated to 3 or 4 cm.[20]

Route of administration. The same drug often can be given by a variety of routes, including intravenous, intramuscular, oral, rectal, and inhalation. Choosing one route over another may help achieve the desired therapeutic response. However, it may also predispose to more pronounced adverse effects if given, for example, by the intravenous route as opposed to the intramuscular route. Dosage adjustments may be necessary when the route of administration is changed.

Combined effects of drugs. Some drugs possess properties similar or identical to drugs of different therapeutic categories. Individually their side effects may be slight, but when combined, the adverse effects may be additive to the point where they are clinically expressed. Effects of some drugs are overadditive (or synergistic) so that the combined effects are greater than predicted by simply adding the two individual effects. Barbiturates, when combined with alcohol, produce a synergistic CNS depression that has led to fatal outcome in nonobstetrical applications.[21]

Although it is unlikely that truly synergistic combinations will be encountered during labor and birth, simple additive side effects are common. A woman receiving one drug for anxiety, one for nausea, and one for pain could easily experience drowsiness contributed by each agent. The combined effects will influence the fetus as well as the mother.

Gestational age. Infants born prematurely often have respiratory difficulties at birth and drugs that depress respiration may aggravate this condition. Also, immature liver and kidney function may preclude efficient handling of drugs. Premature infants are generally more susceptible to drug effects than full-term infants.[22]

Determining the Safety of Obstetrical Drugs

The development of a pharmaceutical product in the United States proceeds according to a plan developed by Congress and carried out under the auspices of the Food and Drug Administration (FDA). There is a logical progression from research studies of relatively low risk to those conducted under actual or near-actual conditions of use. Usually drugs are discovered in the laboratories of pharmaceutical companies, and literally thousands of compounds are screened in laboratory animals to see whether they have any desired drug effects. Before the drug can ever be administered to humans, it must have successfully completed certain segments of FDA's Animal Reproduction Studies. These preclinical reproduction studies are arranged in three parts: (1) single-generation reproduction, (2) teratogenesis, and (3) prenatal-postnatal development. Segment three examines drug effects on late fetal development, labor, delivery, lactation, and newborn health.[23]

Drug research in pregnant women is limited (and rightly so) by moral, legal, and ethical considerations. Double-blind, placebo-controlled study methodologies cannot be employed when the effects of a drug are not known. It would seem unacceptable to give a woman in labor a test dose of a particular drug just to see what might happen to the mother or her fetus. Yet, how is a drug ever proved to be "safe" for obstetrical use? The answer lies in the fact that drugs are often used during pregnancy, labor, and delivery without ever being tested for safety and efficacy, and hence they are actually "tested" in the course of clinical use. Indeed, most data about drug use in human pregnancy are derived from therapeutic use in the clinical environment or are extrapolated from animal studies. But as newer and more potent drugs become available, this process seems less and less acceptable. Essentially, under this logic individual patients given drugs for "therapeutic" purposes are acutally "subjects" in a type of experimental protocol.

Drugs Used During Labor and Delivery

Drug therapy for the perinatal patient can be divided into two broad types, based on the intended purpose and when they are given. Agents given during the first stage of labor are administered to decrease discomfort and relieve anxiety. Drugs given just prior to, or during, the second stage of labor are intended to make the delivery easier by relieving pain and increasing the woman's ability to contribute voluntary effort to give birth. Drugs used during these two periods may be distinctly different or they may be the same drug, varying only in dosage, route, or time of administration.

As stated previously, it is very important that no drug be given which will interfere with the labor process itself. For example, narcotic analgesics such as meperidine (Demerol) may arrest labor if given prior to the establishment of good contractions. A good rule-of-thumb suggests that no sedatives or analgesics be given before a woman has demonstrated positive signs of progressive dilatation and effacement of the cervix. In general, women having their first child should not be administered sedative or analgesic drugs before the cervix is 3 cm dilated, whereas those having their second or subsequent child should not receive these agents until 4 cm of cervical dilatation.

As just noted, the route of administration of obstetrical medication is an important factor to consider. When rapid onset of action is desired, the intravenous route is preferred. However, the dose is usually reduced when the route is selected. The intramuscular route is chosen when a longer duration is desirable. Oral medications are generally not recommended because of the slow and erratic absorption by this route and also because food and liquids are usually withheld during labor.

As with any drug that has sedative properties, the patient should not be left unattended until the full effects of the drug are assessed. This is especially important when the intravenous route is employed because of the more intense effects possible by this route. It is important that intravenous analgesics or sedatives are administered slowly, usually diluted in saline solution or some other intravenous fluid. This permits more careful control and assessment of a patient's response to the drug. If the mother has a "coach" or other attendant during labor, he or she should be instructed about what to look for in terms of side effects and must be encouraged to report suspected drug effects to the nurse or physician.

Narcotic Analgesics

The term "narcotic" is usually applied to a group of analgesic drugs derived from the opium poppy or derivatives produced therefrom. Some narcotics are produced synthetically, but their chemical structure resembles that of the opium alkaloids. Morphine is generally considered the prototype narcotic, and other agents in this category are usually compared with it. Table I lists common narcotic analgesics used in obstetrical practice.

As a class, the narcotics are considered excellent pain relievers. The mechanism by which this is accomplished is poorly understood, but it has been found that the pain-perception threshold is raised, especially when narcotics are administered before the pain is induced.[24] Unfortunately, maternal and neonatal side effects can occur as doses are increased, and, at least theoretically, there is a dose at which an average patient will achieve maximum pain relief with the least number of side effects.[25]

When individual agents are compared, several things become apparent: (1) There is no narcotic that will completely eradicate pain in all patients; (2) used in equianalgesic doses, the degree of pain relief obtained with the various narcotics is similar; and (3) all narcotics have the ability to depress the mother and especially the baby.[22]

Narcotics produce a number of maternal side effects, the most common of which are nausea, vomiting, and dizziness. These effects can be particularly distressing to a woman in labor and may aggravate the nausea that may normally accompany the labor process. Sometimes antinauseant drugs such as promethazine (Phenergan) or hydroxyzine (Vistaril) are combined with narcotics with variable success.

All narcotics have the potential to depress maternal respirations—an effect considered to be the most dangerous acute effect of these drugs.[19] Generally speaking, the respiratory depressant effects are dose related, and at equianalgesic doses the effects are the same.[19] Normal obstetrical doses do not significantly depress maternal respirations, but they may do so in the presence of underlying diseases or if narcotics are combined with other respiratory depressants. Clinically, drug-induced respiratory depression is characterized by slow, irregular, periodic respirations and generally peaks 30 to 90 minutes after parenteral administration.

Narcotics, at concentrations representative of those used in obstetrics, produce no change in contractility of human uterine muscle strips.[26] In practice, however, if the drugs are given too early (that is, the latent phase of the first stage of labor), there is a tendency to slow cervical dilatation, even resulting in uterine inertia.[27] Likewise, excessive doses may interfere with the normal progress of labor. An optimum dose given after 4 to 5 cm of

TABLE I - Narcotic and Narcotic-Like Analgesics Used in Obstetrics

Drug	Brand Name	Dose I.V.	Dose I.M.[a]	Peak Analgesic Effect I.V.	Peak Analgesic Effect I.M.	Duration
Morphine		2-3mg	5-10mg	20 min	60-120 min	4-6 hours
Meperidine	Demerol[R]	25-50mg	50-100mg	5-10 min	40-50 min	3-4 hours
Alphaprodine	Nisentil[R]	10-20mg	30-60mg(sub.q)	1-2 min	5-10 min	1-2 hours
Pentazocine	Talwin[R]	10-20mg	20-30mg	2-3 min	10-20 min	3-4 hours
Fentanyl	Sublimaze[R]	0.025mg-0.05mg	0.05mg-0.1mg	3-5 min	30 min	1-2 hours

[a] alphaprodine should not be administered intramuscularly because of unpredictable absorption.

dilatation will usually have no effect on uterine activity and may even enhance labor by reducing the fear and anxiety that can inhibit the labor process.

Some women receiving narcotics may experience pronounced orthostatic hypotension or lowered blood pressure accompanying sudden changes in posture. This explains the light-headedness or faintness women experience when trying to sit or stand after receiving a narcotic while lying flat. This effect, common to all narcotics, is caused by vasodilation and peripheral pooling of blood. Hypotension is minimal or absent as long as the woman is supine, but parturients who have received narcotics should not be made to walk around because of the risk of fainting.

All narcotics in clinical use cross the placenta in appreciable amounts soon after intravenous injection to the mother, and all exert a direct depressant effect on the respiratory center of the infant. Once placental transfer has occurred, the fetal/neonatal response to most drugs is qualitatively similar to the maternal response. However, the sensitivity of the infant to the depressant effects of drugs is greater in the newborn than at any other time of life.[28] The sensitivity of the mother to narcotic effects does not predict the condition of the infant at birth.[28]

Although mothers may also experience respiratory depression from narcotics, the consequences to the neonate are more ominous than they are in the adult. If respiratory depression is so significant that onset of spontaneous respirations is delayed, the child may soon become acidotic and, if delayed long enough, may suffer permanent brain damage. Although some authors claim that certain narcotics are more or less potent respiratory depressants than others, many firmly contend that the degree of neonatal depression caused by all narcotics during their peak action is about the same when given to the mother in equianalgesic doses.[22]

Depressant effects on the infant are influenced greatly by the timing and route of administration, and some authors feel this is more important than even the amount of the drug given.[28] Following intramuscular administration, the peak depressant effect on the newborn is generally seen during the second and third hour after the dose is given.[22,29] This is true not only for the prototype, morphine, but also for meperidine, methadone, heroin, and dihydrocodeine.[28] With intravenous administration, onset of pain relief is almost immediate, but so are the depressant effects on the child. The dose of intravenous narcotics must be reduced accordingly.

Babies born prematurely have a higher degree of respiratory depression following narcotic administration.[19] The greater the degree of prematurity, the greater is this effect.[30] If a woman is in labor prematurely, it is a good practice to avoid depressant drugs whenever possible.

Narcotics impose a number of effects on the neonate that may not be detectable using gross measures of well-being, such as counting the number of respirations or assessing the vigor of the baby's cry. Even biochemical indices such as maternal and fetal blood levels of drug, pH, and PCO_2, may not totally reflect the more subtle effects of some drugs. Increasingly, investigators are realizing that obstetrical medications can adversely affect infant behavior. Infant assessment by measures more sensitive than the Apgar score has revealed significant narcotic-induced depression in newborns who were otherwise evaluated as normal. Rosen and co-workers[31] demonstrated that 50 mg of meperidine given to women in labor produced subtle changes in fetal and neonatal electroencephalograms (EEG). Brackbill,[32] in her review of obstetrical drugs and their effects on infant behavior, cites numerous studies that show analgesics, principally meperidine, to be harmful to newborn well-being. Effects have been demonstrated on the Brazelton and Scanlon test scores, as well as on mother-infant interaction. Meperidine has been known to depress the habituation to auditory stimuli when doses were given to mothers in labor.[33] This highly sensitive measure of central nervous system functioning was shown to be affected in the face of ''normal'' overall assessment of well-being, adding further to the evidence that drug effects may have escaped detection because the measures used previously have been too gross.[32]

Narcotic antagonists are drugs that compete with narcotics for the pharmacological site of action and whose activity opposes effects seen with these analgesics. There is evidence that narcotic antagonists can reverse the neonatal depressant effects resulting from inappropriate narcotic administration during labor. Naloxone, the favored narcotic antagonist, has been shown to improve ventilation and response to carbon dioxide when given to mothers who had received 1.0 to 1.5 mg/kg of meperidine intravenously 1 hour before vaginal delivery.[28] Similarly, naloxone has been shown to improve neurobehavioral assessments when given to babies passively receiving narcotics.[34] There is little rationale for giving naloxone or any other narcotic antagonist concurrently with the narcotic because it negates any beneficial effect of the pain killer.

General Anesthesia

In the past, general anesthesia was used routinely in those women who wished to know nothing at all of their childbirth experience. It was fashionable in the late nineteenth century to receive heavy sedation and general anesthesia for routine vaginal delivery,[35] and the attitude of "wake me up when it's over" generally prevailed. With today's appreciation of the effects of drugs on infant outcome, it is now considered inappropriate to use general anesthesia for routine vaginal delivery, and except in a certain few instances, general anesthetic techniques are reserved for operative[28] or for complicated vaginal deliveries.

General anesthesia implies loss of sensation throughout the entire body, and agents are administered by either inhalation or intravenous injection. Classically, general anesthetics affect the central nervous system in a progressive fashion; at lower doses analgesia results, proceeding to delirium, surgical anesthesia, and finally respiratory paralysis as doses are increased. Also occurring with dosage increases are adverse effects on the circulatory system, most notably depression of the myocardium and peripheral vessels. Thus "good" anesthesia occurs when desirable central nervous system effects are delicately balanced with other adverse effects on maternal or neonatal physiology.

Suffice it to say that all general anesthetic agents cross the placenta and appear in fetal circulation. The rate and extent to which the individual agents penetrate into the fetal environment vary, but all have the potential to cause neonatal depression. Agents with greater fat solubility tend to cross the placenta more rapidly and seem to enter the central nervous system of both mother and child more easily. It is this attribute which differentiates one anesthetic from another, thereby defining the rapidity of induction of anesthesia and the recovery period once the procedure has been completed.

Neonatal depression is dependent on the concentration of anesthetic present in the newborn's blood at the time of birth. Concentrations described as analgesic (or subanesthetic) generally do not affect the newborn, regardless of duration of use. However, anesthetic concentrations may lead to depression, and the degree of depression depends on both concentration *and* duration of anesthesia.[28]

1. Inhalation Agents

There are several gaseous anesthetics available for use in obstetrics (Table II). One of these, cyclopropane, is experiencing decreasing usage, mainly because it is highly explosive and hence requires special precautions to prevent possible injury. It will be omitted from discussion. Some agents are used prior to surgical delivery (e.g., nitrous oxide), whereas others (e.g., halothane) are often reserved for the portion of surgery occurring after the baby has been delivered.

Nitrous oxide. Popular as an analgesic/anesthetic in dental practice,

Table II - General Anesthetics Used in Obstetrics

Agent	Brand Name	Analgesic Dose	Anesthetic Dose
Inhalation Anesthetics			
Isoflurane	Forane[R]	0.2 - 0.7%	0.5 - 3%[a]
Halothane	Fluothane[R]	_____	0.5 - 1.5%[a]
Enflurane	Ethrane[R]	0.25 - 1.25%	1.5 - 3.0%[a]
Methoxyflurane	Penthrane[R]	0.3 - 0.6%	0.1 - 2.0%[b]
Nitrous Oxide	_____	50 - 70%	50 - 70%
Injectable Anesthetics			
Ketamine	Ketalar, Ketaject[R]	5 - 10 mg[c]	1 - 2 mg/kg
Thiopental	Pentothal[R]	_____	_____

[a]Lower concentrations are used when combined with nitrous oxide.

[b]When combined with at least 50% nitrous oxide in oxygen.

[c]Total dose given intermittently.

nitrous oxide, sometimes referred to as "laughing gas," is perhaps the most frequently used inhalation anesthetic in obstetrical practice. Below a concentration of 50% of inspired air, nitrous oxide is considered analgesic, since the patient remains conscious and can participate in the birth process. Consequently, nitrous oxide is frequently used during the second stage of labor to calm an agitated patient. Fetal levels of nitrous oxide are achieved rapidly, and after 3 to 4 minutes of anesthesia, have reached levels eight tenths that in maternal blood. At higher concentrations given to the mother, neonatal depression can occur as a result of high fetal brain concentrations.[36] In the past, serious fetal damage occurred when 100% or nearly 100% nitrous oxide mixture was used, thus preventing oxygen from reaching the mother. The mother, and particularly the infant, suffered the effects of oxygen deprivation. Today, nitrous oxide is usually administered along with oxygen in a ratio of 70 to 30 nitrous oxide to oxygen, and if used for a reasonable length of time, produces little depression on the newborn.

Methoxyflurane. This volatile agent is more frequently used as a self-administered analgesic in the first stage of labor than as a general anesthetic. Among other forms, it is packaged in a unique "whistle" similar to a flute a child might use. At the height of a uterine contraction, the patient is instructed to take a few whiffs of the gas to help relieve discomfort. This analgesia is usually well tolerated—indeed, patients should be closely observed to dissuade excessive use.

Methoxyflurane has lost favor as a general anesthetic because of reported cases of renal toxicity.[28] However, Rosen and associates[37] studied the use of this drug during labor and were unable to detect impairment of renal function. Based on studies of the metabolism of methoxyflurane, Fry and Taves[38] concluded that exposure to this drug, even at anesthetic concentrations, is probably safe in the obstetrical patient if the duration of administration does not exceed 30 minutes.

Halothane. This gaseous anesthetic produces a relaxant effect on the uterus and therefore is not normally used during labor. In instances where relaxation becomes necessary (that is, mechanical extraction of a breech baby when the cervix clamps around the infant's neck), halothane is often effective in overcoming the complication.

Halothane is used in low concentration combined with nitrous oxide, allowing smaller concentrations of nitrous oxide to be used. The net result permits higher concentrations of oxygen to be used while achieving acceptable surgical anesthesia.

Albert and associates[39] have reported a high frequency of postpartum hemorrhage following nitrous oxide–oxygen–halothane anesthesia. Presumably this effect can be attributed to the uterine relaxant properties of halothane, resulting in postpartum atony and hemorrhage.

Enflurane. This halogenated ether is widely used to induce general anesthesia and, unlike halothane, it has considerable analgesic properties when given in low doses. However, enflurane shares halothane's ability to relax the uterus, and doses of 3% or more may result in uterine atony.[40] As with halothane, enflurane rapidly crosses the placenta and enters the fetal circulation. Both anesthetics are detectable in the umbilical vein blood within 2 minutes after administration to the mother.[41] When low concentrations (0.5%) are used to decrease maternal awareness during cesarean section, enflurane is not associated with neonatal depressant effects.[28] Coleman and Downing[42] reported a series of 50 parturients anesthetized with enflurane (0.5% to 0.8% before cesarean delivery and 1.0% to 1.5% after the baby was delivered), and in none of the infants was there evidence of perinatal depression. As with halothane, enflurane allows use of smaller amounts of nitrous oxide, thus permitting increased oxygen concentrations in inspired gas.[43]

Isoflurane. This is the latest nonflammable inhalation anesthetic to become commercially available in the United States. Chemically, isoflurane is nearly identical to enflurane. Its low lipid solubility allows rapid induction and recovery from anesthesia. Some patients find the odor of isoflurane to be disagreeably pungent. In keeping with halothane and enflurane, isoflurane causes a dose-dependent depression of myometrial contractility.[44]

When given at very high doses, isoflurane decreases maternal blood pressure and cardiac output, which causes decreased uterine blood flow with resultant fetal hypoxia and acidosis. Light or moderate anesthesia with isoflurane produces no readily discernible untoward effects on the fetus.[45]

Because clinical experience with isoflurane in obstetrics is limited,[45] particularly when used during complicated vaginal delivery or cesarean section, perhaps it is best to select an alternative agent for which more definitive data are available.

2. Injectable Analgesic/Anesthetics

Two injectable anesthetics are commonly employed in obstetrics, namely thiopental (Sodium Pentothal) and ketamine. Thiopental is used mainly for induction of anesthesia rather than maintenance, whereas ketamine is used in higher doses for induction and at lower doses for analgesia and amnesia.

Thiopental. Thiopental is a rapidly acting barbiturate that owes its quick onset and short duration to an extremely high lipid solubility. Within 1 minute after intravenous injection, thiopental crosses the placental and maternal blood-brain barrier.[46] If no other drugs are given, the duration of anesthesia is 10 minutes after a single bolus injection.[46]

Because thiopental can depress contractility of the heart and because it can cause a peripheral vasodilation, hypotension can become a problem. Thiopental is seldom used as a sole anesthetic in obstetrics but is frequently used to induce the anesthetic state rapidly.

Ketamine. Ketamine has potent amnesic and analgesic properties and has been used as an alternative to thiopental as an induction agent. Combined with nitrous oxide, ketamine is also used as a general anesthetic for cesarean section.[47] Uterine blood flow actually improves with ketamine administration,[48] and effects on uterine contractility are dose dependent: Minimal changes are associated with low doses (1.1 mg/kg) and greater changes accompany larger doses (2.2 mg/kg).[49]

Ketamine crosses the placenta rapidly, but if doses are kept at or below 1 mg/kg, fetal depression is unlikely.[50] However, as doses are increased above 2 mg/kg, a high rate of neonatal depression is seen.[50]

In small doses (0.25 mg/kg) ketamine is used during labor for analgesia and amnesia.[46] It is sometimes used in conjunction with epidural and spinal anesthesia when inadequate pain relief is obtained by these procedures alone.

Because ketamine is structurally related to the psychomimetic drug phencyclidine (PCP), it shares some of the adverse effects of the latter drug. In fact, in one study[51] over 30% of patients experienced unpleasant dreams or hallucinations—an effect that makes ketamine less satisfactory than thiopental for induction of anesthesia for elective cesarean section.

Newborn Outcome With General Anesthesia

Studies focusing on Apgar scores at birth have shown that there are more depressed infants at 1 minute with general anesthesia than with regional anesthesia; by the 5-minute mark, however, Apgar scores are virtually identical for both techniques. By the 5-minute mark, the baby has "blown off" anesthetic gas and the transient drug-related depression has cleared.[52] Significant newborn depression seems to be associated with unusually long durations of general anesthesia. Stenger and co-workers[53] found a 15% incidence of newborn depression after 15 minutes of nitrous oxide anesthesia, with the incidence of depression rising to 54% after 36 minutes.

Anesthetic-related neonatal depression is better measured by more subtle neurobehavioral tests than by gross measures such as Apgar score. Scanlon and associates[54] reported that cesarean infants were more depressed 8 hours after general anesthesia than infants delivered under spinal anesthesia when measured using the Scanlon neurobehavioral scale. Others have reported similar findings.[52] The long-term significance of these findings is uncertain.

Regional Anesthesia

Women are increasingly electing to be "awake and aware" during the birth of their children. Regional anesthesia, or the use of local anesthetics to cause loss of sensations in limited areas of the body, allows the parturient to remain conscious throughout the delivery process and to provide the much needed cooperation to expedite delivery of the baby. Furthermore, the use of regional anesthesia affords a degree of freedom from the depressant effects of drugs on the fetus. Even during cesarean section many women wish to be fully conscious as events proceed.

Although the drugs used in the various types of regional anesthesia may be the same (Table III), the site of administration affects the quality of the anesthesia and risks involved. Techniques range from a simple infiltration of local anesthetic into the perineal area to injecting into the subarachnoid space of the spinal column.

Local infiltration of the perineum. This technique involves injection of

Table III - Local Anesthetics Used in Obstetrics

Drug	Brand Name	Classification
Lidocaine	Xylocaine[R]	Amide
Mepivacaine	Carbocaine[R]	Amide
Bupivacaine	Marcaine[R]	Amide
Etidocaine	Duranest[R]	Amide
Prilocaine	Citanest[R]	Amide
Procaine	Novocaine[R]	Ester
Chloroprocaine	Nesacaine[R]	Ester
Tetracaine	Pontocaine[R]	Ester

a suitable local anesthetic agent into several locations surrounding the vaginal opening. Although satisfactory for cutting and repairing the episiotomy, this technique provides little relief for the pain sensations arising from the uterus and cervix. For this reason, local infiltration is used infrequently as a single anesthetic agent.

Pudendal block. Pudendal block involves blocking nerve impulses carried by the pudendal nerve, a large nerve carrying impulses from the perineum, the clitoris, and the rectal area. By injecting a local anesthetic agent into the pudendal nerve, pain impulses are prevented from reaching the spinal cord. In effect, the perineum is numbed and pain arising from the stretching, dilating, and distention of the vaginal outlet and perineum can be completely eliminated.[55]

Some skill is required to administer pudendal block anesthesia correctly, but the risks from this technique are low. The most notable maternal risk is failure to achieve adequate analgesia. The intensity of the uterine contractions is not affected,[56] nor is there interference with the mother's ability to bear down with contractions. If the drug is inadvertently injected into an artery or vein, systemic toxic reactions can occur. Simple precautions before the drug is injected can almost always prevent this from happening.

Although some local anesthetic injected into the pudendal nerve can appear in the fetal circulation, few adverse effects attributable to this technique have been reported.

Paracervical anesthesia. Much of the pain associated with labor is caused by dilatation of the cervix. Pain pathways that originate in the cervix can be interrupted by the injection of local anesthetic around the outside of the cervix at the cervical-uterine junction. This technique is particularly used during the active phase of the first stage of labor, when cervical dilatation is at 4 to 6 cm.[57]

Using a hollow needle guide, the drug is injected into several locations (usually 2 to 4) around the cervical area. Although pain relief is rapid, the duration of effect is usually short. Depending on which agent is used, pain relief will usually last for 45 to 60 minutes with 1% lidocaine, whereas 2% 2-chloroprocaine lasts only 30 to 45 minutes.[58] Thus throughout the course of a long labor, several readministrations may be necessary. As will be shown, toxicity occurs as the total dose increases.

Most women tolerate paracervical anesthesia well. As with pudendal block, inadvertent injection into a blood vessel can produce systemic effects such as palpitations, tinnitus, metallic taste, drowsiness, confusion, loss of consciousness, convulsions, hypotension, and slowed heart rate. Fortunately, these effects are rare and are usually transient in nature when they do occur.[57]

Fetal complications, on the other hand, are more frequent and more severe. Fetal bradycardia has been reported in from 2% to 70% of newborns of mothers receiving paracervical anesthesia.[57] Changes in fetal heart rate are usually detected within 2 to 10 minutes after injection. The exact cause of the bradycardia is not known, but the leading theories include (1) a decrease in uterine blood flow, (2) the direct depressant effects on fetal myocardium, or (3) depression of the fetal central nervous system. High fetal levels of local anesthetic are associated with bradycardia. The fetal bradycardia may lead to acidosis resulting from hypoxemia of the infant. This effect is most often seen when the bradycardia extends beyond 10 minutes. Apgar scores of infants born during post-paracervical bradycardia are consistently lower than in babies delivered at times other than during a bradycardic episode.[59] Resuscitative measures may be necessary if fetal distress is severe. Prolonged bradycardia (beyond 20 minutes) is an ominous sign and has been the cause of perinatal deaths.[60] Continuous electronic fetal monitoring is essential whenever paracervical block analgesia is used.

Caudal epidural anesthesia. This technique involves injection of a local anesthetic into the caudal canal at the base of the spinal column by way of a needle or plastic catheter inserted into the canal. The anesthetic is injected into the space outside the spinal cord and blocks impulses as the nerves emerge from the cord. With the catheter in place, repeated injections of local anesthetic allow a continuous blockade.

Maternal complications include hypotension, inadvertent intravenous injection, and accidental puncture of the dura which results in a total spinal anesthesia. The effect of caudal anesthesia on the progress of labor is variable, depending on the degree of cervical dilatation, frequency and intensity of uterine contractions, and the amount and type of anesthetic used.[61] If administered before active labor is established or if it is combined with large doses of sedatives or analgesics, labor is most likely to be delayed.

The local anesthetic blocks pain sensations carried via the sacral nerves and anesthetizes the pelvis. When successful, the woman in labor experiences no pain, but she is not conscious of uterine contractions. It can be used as an analgesic in the first and second stages of labor and as an anesthetic for delivery.

Lumbar epidural anesthesia. This local anesthetic is also injected into the space outside the lining of the spinal column. However, this technique involves injecting in the space between the second lumbar vertebra and the first sacral vertebra. The technique of lumbar epidural is technically easier than caudal anesthesia, the failure rate is lower, and smaller amounts of local anesthetic are required.

As is the case with caudal epidural anesthesia, the most common maternal complication is hypotension, occurring in from 1.4% to 12% of women.[62] This occurs because of blockage of sympathetic impulses, resulting in a consequent loss of peripheral vascular resistance. To prevent a disastrous outcome for both the mother and fetus, vital signs should be taken frequently during administration of epidural anesthesia. If the systolic blood pressure falls below 100 mm Hg or greater than 30% of the preanesthetic pressure, treatment to reverse this process must be undertaken.[63] When maternal hypotension occurs, the fetus is also affected by virtue of decreased perfusion of blood to the uterus. Changes in the fetal heart rate patterns indicative of uteroplacental insufficiency are often associated with maternal hypotension during epidural block.[64]

The intensity of uterine contractions may be decreased by the use of epidural anesthesia,[57] but great debate surrounds the frequency and predisposing factors associated with this adverse effect.

Lumbar epidural anesthesia can be given as a one-time injection, or a catheter can be inserted for continuous anesthesia. When small doses are used, pain relief adequate for labor is obtained. Increasing doses are given as delivery becomes imminent.

Large doses, often referred to as surgical anesthesia, produce anesthesia suitable for operative delivery. More and more women are choosing this technique in an effort to participate more actively or at least be aware of the events surrounding cesarean delivery.

Spinal anesthesia. With spinal anesthesia, local anesthetic is injected into the cerebrospinal fluid in the subarachnoid space below the level of the spinal cord. Smaller doses are suitable for vaginal delivery, whereas larger doses produce anesthesia for cesarean section. Variations in techniques of positioning the patient after injection result in either complete spinal anesthesia or "saddle block" anesthesia, whereby anesthesia of only the perineum is produced. The advantage of the saddle block lies in the fact that women are more capable of bearing down when only the perineum is blocked, but pain relief may be incomplete with this technique.

Hodgkinson and associates[65] have shown that neonates delivered by elective cesarean section under spinal anesthesia had higher scores on neurobehavioral tests than a comparable group delivered under general anesthesia. Spinal anesthesia does not appear to affect the force of uterine contractions significantly.[59] However, when complete spinal anesthesia is employed, the woman's inability to bear down effectively may cause an increase in the length of the second stage of labor, requiring increased use of forceps to effect delivery.

Maternal hypotension is the most serious complication with spinal anesthesia. The incidence is relatively low when spinal anesthesia is used for vaginal birth (saddle block) and is high (up to 92%) with spinal anesthesia for operative delivery.[66]

Another maternal complication of spinal anesthesia is the so-called "spinal headache," which is thought to result from leakage of spinal fluid through the site of puncture into the spinal membranes.[67] A unique feature of this headache is that the pain occurs or is worsened when the head is raised and goes away or is reduced in intensity when the woman lies down. Symptoms usually appear the day after the spinal anesthesia and typically disappear 5 to 6 days later.[58] The frequency and severity of postspinal headaches are related to needle size used during the technique; the use of a 20-gauge needle results in an incidence of headache in 41% of women, whereas using a 24-gauge needle drops the rate of occurrence to 0.4%.[68] Whenever possible a small needle should be used.

Patient Rights and Responsibilities

Women in labor sometimes are reluctant to ask questions concerning medications they are about to receive. They feel powerless to refuse medications or to inquire about side effects, dosages, or other important facts. But childbearing women not only have the right but also the responsibility to know as much as possible, good and bad, about drugs they may receive. Infant well-being may depend on the competency of the mother's decision-making abilities. The following suggestions may help expectant parents plan and manage their drug therapy during labor and birth.

Role of drugs. Some couples, especially those attending prepared childbirth classes, have the mistaken notion that if they receive drugs during labor they have somehow failed themselves or their instructor. Nothing could be more untrue; drugs sometimes can make the difference between a pleasant, positive childbirth experience and a disastrous one. Childbirth classes do emphasize keeping drugs to a minimum, but most importantly, they teach the couple to make informed choices. No one fails at childbirth, especially when the woman lets her wishes be known.

Planning the drug therapy. It is most important that expectant parents discuss drug options with the obstetrician before going to the hospital. Research shows that patients in the hospital environment relinquish decision making to others,[69] and furthermore, the clamor of a busy labor suite is an unsuitable environment for discussing drugs.

All available alternatives should be presented, not just those preferred by the physician. Undoubtedly, the practitioner will have his or her favorite technique, but if it is not acceptable to the patient for any reason, by all means she should let this be known. For example, some women cannot bear the thought of a needle being inserted into the back; for them epidural anesthesia is a poor choice.

The woman should ask what drugs are available to relieve the discomfort of labor, treat nausea or vomiting, reduce anxiety, and ease birth. Some long labors may require a period of rest; sleeping medications are generally not necessary, but one should nevertheless inquire about these drugs. Couples should ask also about techniques for anesthesia should complications necessitate cesarean delivery.

It may be desirable to have drug orders written in advance, with instructions to institute therapy only when requested by the patient. In this manner, orders are individualized according to the patient's needs and desires. Standing orders, a preprinted set of physician's directives to be carried out in his or her absence, usually call for automatic administration of a fixed dose of a drug in a "cookbook" fashion. This approach should be discouraged. Patients are not all alike—they vary according to height, weight, tolerance to pain, and many other factors. Drugs and dosages appropriate for a 165-pound woman are clearly excessive for a patient weighing 105 pounds. Some women go through labor without needing any medications, whereas others require several drugs. Standing orders do not acknowledge the individuality of the childbearing woman.

In discussing drugs with the obstetrician, the woman should focus on the drug itself, its route of administration, the dosage, and the timing of its administration as labor progresses. If not satisfied with the explanation, she should ask that it be explained again, perhaps in a slightly different way. Expectant parents should keep asking questions until they are satisfied with their understanding of the drug's effects. Patients are paying their doctors for what they know and therefore are entitled to share in this knowledge.

Labor and birth. Most labor and delivery personnel are happy to accommodate an expectant couple's reasonable desires during the childbirth experience. Some, however, are still practicing in the days when patients were kept in the dark about procedures to be done or drugs to be given. Personnel may try to dictate what drugs the woman needs and when she needs them. In fact, some will even withhold the name of a drug about to be given. This should not be tolerated by today's childbearing parents. An expectant mother has the right to know what the nurse proposes to give her, its dose, and any side effects that can be expected. She should not accept vague explanations like, "It's something for pain" or "It's something to make you more comfortable." She must insist on knowing all she can about what is in the syringe which is about to be stuck into her. If she is not completely satisfied with the explanations or if she feels the risks are too high, it must be remembered that *a patient has the right to refuse any medications* she does not want to receive.

In the foregoing context, the patient must be assertive. Unfortunately, during labor a woman is vulnerable and may yield to pressure from the labor and delivery staff. If she feels that her desires are being ignored, she should ask to speak directly with the obstetrician. Because of earlier planning, the physician already knows her feelings about drugs and is in a position to reinforce her preferences. The worst thing would be for a woman to yield to the pressure to use a drug just to make someone else happy or to avoid a commotion. With careful advance planning this problem can be avoided.

REFERENCES

1. Snow J. *On chloroform and other anaesthetics: Their action and administration.* pp XXXI+19, London, John Churchill, 1858. (Reprinted by the American Society of Anesthesiologists, Chicago, 1950.)

2. Moya F, Thorndike V. Passage of drugs across the placenta. *Am J Obstet Gynecol* 84:1778–1798, 1962.

3. Levhoff AH. Perinatal outcome of paroxysmal tachycardia of the newborn with onset in utero. *Am J Obstet Gynecol* 104:73–79, 1969.

4. Idanpaan-Heikkla JE, Jouppila PI, Puolakka JO, et al. Placental transport and fetal metabolism of diazepam in early human pregnancy. *Am J Obstet Gynecol* 109:1011–1016, 1971.

5. Hellman LM, Pritchard JA. *Williams Obstetrics* (14th ed) New York, Appleton-Century-Crofts, 1971.

6. Eckenhoff JE, Oech SR. The effects of narcotics and antagonists upon respiration and circulation in man. *Clin Pharmacol Ther* 1:483–524, 1960.

7. Friedman EA, Sachtleben MR, Wallace AK. Infant outcome following labor induction. *Am J Obstet Gynecol* 133:718–722, 1979.

8. Rane A, Wilson JT. Clinical pharmacokinetics in infants and children. *Clin Pharmacokinet* 1:2–24, 1976.

9. Rubin MI, Bruck E, Rapoport MJ. Maturation of renal function in childhood: Clearance studies. *Clin Invest* 28:1144, 1949.

10. Morrison JC, Whiprew WD, Rosser SI, et al. Metabolites of meperidine in the fetal and maternal serum. *Am J Obstet Gynecol* 126:997–1002, 1976.

11. Reynolds SRM, Harris JS, Kaiser IH. *Clinical measurement of uterine forces in pregnancy and labor.* Springfield, IL, Charles C Thomas, Publisher, 1954.

12. Dobbing J, Sands J. Quantitative growth and development of human brain. *Arch Dis Child* 48:757–767, 1973.

13. Hughes JG, Hill FS, Green CR, et al. Electroencephalography of the newborn V: Brain potentials of babies born of mothers given meperidine hydrochloride (Demerol hydrochloride), vinbarbital sodium (Delvinal sodium) or morphine. *Am J Dis Child* 79:996–1007, 1950.

14. Brackbill Y, Kane J, Manniello RL, et al. Obstetrical meperidine usage and assessment of neonatal status. *Anesthesiology* 40:116–120, 1974.

15. Brower KR. Effects of intranatal drugs on the newborn EEG. Unpublished MA Thesis, University of Hawaii, 1974.

16. Aleksandrowicz MK, Aleksandrowicz DR. Obstetrical pain-relieving drugs as predictors of infant behavior variability. *Child Devel* 45:935–945, 1974.

17. Scanlon JW, Ostheimer GW, Brown WV, et al. Neurobehavioral responses of newborns after epidural anesthesia with bupivacaine. *Anesthesiology* 45:400–405, 1976.

18. Horowitz FD, Ashton J, Culp R, et al. The effects of obstetrical medication on the behavior of Israeli newborn infants and some comparisons with Uruguayan and American infants. *Child Devel* 48:1607–1623, 1977.

19. Bonica JJ. Effects of analgesia and anesthesia on the fetus and newborn. In Caldeyro-Barcia R (ed). *Effects of labor and delivery on the fetus and newborn.* New York, Pergamon Press, 1967.

20. Tuchmann-Duplessis H. *Drug effects on the fetus.* New York, ADIS Press, 1975.

21. Arena JM. *Poisoning: Toxicology, symptoms, treatment* (3rd ed) Springfield, IL, Charles C Thomas, Publisher, 1974.

22. Bonica JJ. *Principles and practice of obstetric analgesia and anesthesia.* Philadelphia, FA Davis Co, 1967.

23. Kinney EL, Trautmann J, Gold JA, et al. Underrepresentation of women in new drug trials. *Ann Int Med* 95:495–499, 1981.

24. French JD, Verzeano M, Magoun HW. A neural basis of the anesthetic state. *Arch Neurol Psychiat* 69:519–529, 1953.

25. Lasagna L, Beecher HK. The optimal dose of morphine. *JAMA* 156:230–234, 1954.

26. Talbert LM, McGaughey HS Jr, Corey EL, et al. Effects of anesthetic and sedative agents commonly employed in obstetric practice on isolated human uterine muscle. *Am J Obstet Gynecol* 75:16–22, 1958.

27. James LS. The effect of pain relief for labor and delivery on the fetus and newborn. *Anesthesiology* 21:405–430, 1960.

28. Bassell GM, Belonsky BL, Marx GF. Systemic anesthetic methods. In Marx GF, Bassell GM (eds). *Obstetric analgesia and anesthesia.* New York, Elsevier North Holland, 1980.

29. McNab JA. Obstetrical analgesia and anaesthesia. *Can Med Assoc J* 72:681–686, 1955.

30. Moya F, Thorndike V. The effects of drugs used in labor on the fetus and newborn. *Clin Pharmacol Ther* 4:628–653, 1963.

31. Rosen MG, Scibetta JJ, Devroude PJ. In Marx GM (ed). *Parturition and perinatology*. Philadelphia, F.A. Davis Co, 1973.

32. Brackbill Y. Obstetrical medication and infant behavior. In Osofsky JD (ed). *The handbook of infant development*. New York, John Wiley & Sons, 1974.

33. Brackbill Y, Kane J, Manniello RL, et al. Obstetrical premedication and infant outcome. *Am J Obstet Gynecol* 118:377–384, 1974.

34. Hodgkinson R, Bhatt M, Grewal G, et al. Neonatal neurobehavior in first 48 hours of life—effect of administration of meperidine with and without naloxone in mother. *Pediatrics* 62:294–298, 1978.

35. DeVore JS. Psychologic analgesia. In Marx GF, Bassell GM (eds). *Obstetrical analgesia and anesthesia*. New York, Elsevier North Holland, 1980.

36. Reid DHS. Diffusion anoxia at birth. *Lancet* 2:757–758, 1968.

37. Rosen M, Latto P, Asscher AW. Kidney function after methoxyflurane analgesia during labor. *Br Med J* 1:81–83, 1972.

38. Fry BW, Taves DR. Maternal and fetal fluorometabolite concentrations after exposure to methoxyflurane. *Am J Obstet Gynecol* 119:199–204, 1974.

39. Albert CA, Anderson G, Wallace W, et al. Fluothane for obstetric anesthesia. *Obstet Gynecol* 13:282–284. 1959.

40. Marx GF, Kim YI, Lim CC, et al. Postpartum uterine pressures under halothane or enflurane anesthesia. *Obstet Gynecol* 51:695–698, 1978.

41. Scheridan CA, Robson JG. Fluothane in obstetrical anaesthesia. *Can Anaesth Soc J* 6:365–374, 1959.

42. Coleman AJ, Downing JW. Ethrane anaesthesia for caesarean section. *S Afr Med J* 49:1927–1929, 1975.

43. Moir DD. Anaesthesia for caesarean section. *Br J Anaesth* 42:136–142, 1970.

44. Munson ES, Embro WJ. Enflurane, isoflurane, and halothane and isolated human uterine muscle. *Anesthesiology* 46:11–14, 1977.

45. Wade JG, Stevens WC. Isoflurane: An anesthetic for the eighties? *Anesth Analg* 60:662–682, 1981.

46. James FM III. Pharmacology of anesthetics. *Clin Obstet Gynecol* 24:561–573, 1981.

47. Hodgkinson R, Marx GF, Kim SS, et al. Neonatal neurobehavioral tests following vaginal delivery under ketamine, thiopental, and extradural anesthesia. *Anesth Analg* 56:548–553, 1977.

48. Levinson G, Shnider SM, Gildea JE, et al. Maternal and fetal cardiovascular and acid-base changes during ketamine anesthesia in pregnant ewes. *Br J Anaesth* 45:1111–1115, 1973.

49. Galloon S. Ketamine for obstetric delivery. *Anesthesiology* 44:522–524, 1976.

50. Janeczko CF, El-Etr AA, Younes SS. Low dose ketamine anesthesia for vaginal delivery. *Anesth Analg* 53:828–831, 1974.

51. Little B, Chang T, Chucot L, et al. Study of ketamine as an obstetric anesthetic agent. *Am J Obstet Gynecol* 113:247–260, 1972.

52. Maduska AL. Inhalation analgesia and general anesthesia. *Clin Obstet Gynecol* 24:619–633, 1981.

53. Stenger VG, Blechmen JN, Prystowsky H. A study of prolongation of obstetric anesthesia. *Am J Obstet Gynecol* 103:901–907, 1969.

54. Scanlon JW, Shea E, Alper MH. Neurobehavioral responses of newborn infants following general or spinal anesthesia for cesarean section. Abstracts of Scientific Papers, Annual Meeting, American Society of Anesthesiologists, Chicago, 1975.

55. Klink EW. Perineal nerve block: An anatomic and clinical study in the female. *Obstet Gynecol* 1:137–146, 1953.

56. Johnson WL, Winter WW, Eng M, et al. Effect of pudendal, spinal and peridural block anesthesia on the second stage of labor. *Am J Obstet Gynecol* 113:166–175, 1972.

57. King JC, Sherline DM. Paracervical and pudendal block. *Clin Obstet Gynecol* 24:587–595, 1981.

58. Fox GS, Morris G. Conduction anesthesia. In Marx GF, Bassell GM (eds). *Obstetrical analgesia and anesthesia*. New York, Elsevier North Holland, 1980.

59. Teramo K. Studies on foetal acid-base values after paracervical blockade during labour. *Acta Obstet Gynecol Scand* 48(suppl 3):80–82, 1969.

60. Rosefsky JB, Petersiel ME. Perinatal deaths associated with mepivacaine paracervical block anesthesia in labor. *N Engl J Med* 287:530–533, 1968.

61. Gottschalk W. Anesthesia in obstetrics, symposium. *Clin Obstet Gynecol* 17(2):139–144, 1974.

62. Caseby NG. Epidural analgesia for the surgical induction of labour. *Br J Anaesth* 46:747–751, 1974.

63. Shnider S, Levinson G. *Anesthesia for obstetrics*. Baltimore, Williams & Wilkins Co, 1979.

64. Schiffrin BS. Fetal heart rate patterns following epidural anaesthesia and oxytocin infusion during labour. *J Obstet Gynaecol Br Commonw* 79:332–339, 1972.

65. Hodgkinson R, Bhatt M, Kim SS, et al. Neonatal neurobehavioral tests following cesarean section under general and spinal anesthesia. *Am J Obstet Gynecol* 132:670–674, 1978.

66. Clark RB, Thompson DS, Thompson CH. Prevention of spinal hypotension associated with cesarean section. *Anesthesiology* 45:670–674, 1976.

67. Crawford JS. The prevention of headache consequent upon dural puncture. *Br J Anaesth* 44:598–600, 1972.

68. Greene BA. A 26 gauge lumbar puncture needle: Its value in the prophylaxis of headache following spinal analgesia for vaginal delivery. *Anesthesiology* 11:464–469, 1950.

69. Waitzkin H, Stoeckle JD. Information control and the micropolitics of health care: Summary of an ongoing research project. *Soc Sci Med* 10:263–276, 1976.

SUBMITTED: JUNE, 1982
REVISED & ACCEPTED: AUGUST, 1982

BENEFITS AND RISKS OF EPISIOTOMY

Stephen B. Thacker
H. David Banta

In recent years the benefits and risks of routinely used medical procedures have been increasingly questioned. Many technologies* were widely used before they were found to have little or no benefit. Such technologies include internal mammary artery ligation for coronary artery disease, lumbodorsal sympathectomy for asthma, and gastric freezing for peptic ulcers.[43] Rising health care costs have focused attention on the issue of appropriate use of medical technology. Routinely used obstetrical interventions, such as electronic fetal monitoring,[3] cesarean section,[49] induction of labor,[21] perineal shaving,[46] and obstetrical anesthesia[13] have been criticized.

Medicine has tended to develop empirically, by trial and error. Methods for the scientific assessment of benefits and risks of technology are still fairly new. More and more, new technology tends to be the subject of carefully controlled clinical trials. However, older "established" technology often has not been examined. We therefore decided to examine the literature on a widely used intervention, episiotomy, which is already controversial.[26,41]

Background

Episiotomy is surgical enlargement of the vaginal orifice during labor and delivery. It is generally done by a midline or mediolateral incision downward toward the anus and can be extended into the rectum[61,73] (Figure 1). Strictly speaking, "episiotomy" refers to surgical cutting of the external genitals. The more accurate term, "perineotomy," refers to making a surgical incision of the perineum, the area between the vulva and the anus. However, following common usage, the procedure will be called episiotomy in this paper.

Episiotomy is done during labor when the baby's head is exposed to a

The authors wish to thank Willard Cates, MD, Iain Chalmers, MB, MRCOG, David Grimes, MD, Doris Haire, Joseph Kahn, MD, Joyce Lashof, MD, Ruth Lubic, CNM, EdD, Herbert L. Peterson, MD, and Norma Swenson, MPH, for their comments and suggestions.

*The drugs, devices, and medical/surgical procedures used in medical care.

161

Fig. I INCISIONS OF MEDIAN AND MEDIOLATERAL EPISIOTOMIES

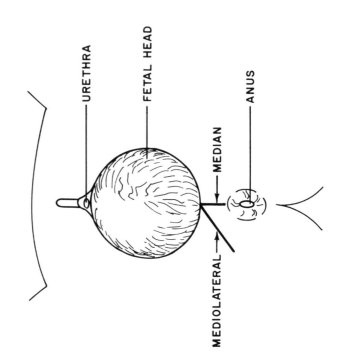

diameter of 3 to 4 cm. If it is done earlier, excessive bleeding can result. If it is done much later, the pelvic tissues will already be considerably stretched. Episiotomy is a necessary part of forceps deliveries or forceps-assisted deliveries, as well as breech presentations and the births of very large babies. Its use in these situations seems well supported by clinical experience, although interventions such as epidural anesthesia can make intervention by forceps and episiotomy necessary.

As a surgical procedure, episiotomy requires repair by suturing (sewing) after the placenta has been delivered. It is generally simple but can be complicated if lacerations (tears) have occurred. Pain often follows episiotomy, and heat lamps, ice, and analgesics are routinely given to relieve such pain.

Williams Obstetrics describes episiotomy as the commonest operation in obstetrics, with the one exception of cutting and tying the umbilical cord.[61] The reasons for episiotomy are stated as follows:

> First, it substitutes a straight, clean surgical incision for the ragged laceration that otherwise frequently results. Furthermore, the episiotomy is easier to repair and heals better than a tear. Second, it spares the baby's head the necessity of serving as a battering ram against perineal obstruction. If prolonged, the poundings of the infant's head against the perineum may cause brain injury. Third, the operation shortens the second stage of labor. Finally, mediolateral episiotomy reduces the likelihood of third-degree lacerations.

Another commonly cited benefit is the preservation of the pelvic floor and perineum by decreasing the pounding of the infant's head on these tissues.[31,39]

The major purpose of this paper is to examine the assertions of that paragraph. Another purpose is to review the risks of episiotomy, which are little discussed in *Williams Obstetrics*.

Historical Perspective

Until the early 1800s, it was uncommon to find a birth attendant who was not a woman and a midwife. However, with developments in scientific medicine in the 1800s, obstetrics began to develop as a medical specialty but was hampered in its growth by the perceived role of the hospital, which was basically a place where poor people went to die. Puerperal fever was frequently caused by obstetricians in carrying out a hospital delivery because of the lack of knowledge regarding sterile technique and the bacterial causes of disease. However, the prevention of puerpural fever became possible in the late 1800s, and the middle class began to accept hospital delivery by obstetricians. At the same time, the midwife began to disappear and was virtually eliminated in the United States by propaganda and legislation during the early 1900s. Obstetricians argued that women were constitutionally unfit to be birth attendants.[5,75]

With the control of infection in hospitals, the location of delivery began to shift. In 1900 fewer than 5% of women in the United States gave birth in hospitals; by the 1950s over 80% of deliveries were done in hospitals. At the same time, modern surgery developed rapidly. The introduction of anesthesia in the early 1900s encouraged the use of surgery.[5] Historically, physicians have been trained to intervene in disease processes. Obstetricians tended to see birth as a dangerous, even pathological process.[29,74]These trends fostered intervention in labor and delivery, which parents accepted because they were having smaller families and hoped that each baby would survive and be healthy.[75]

One of the surgical procedures developed during this period was episiotomy. Ould first described the potential advantages of such a procedure in 1746.[59] At that time, the technique was described as multiple nicks around the vaginal outlet or bilateral cuts perpendicular to the vaginal opening.[48,59] (As described earlier, it now involves one incision.) Braun apparently coined the term "episiotomy," but he believed that the procedure was inadvisable and unnecessary.[58] Taliaferro introduced episiotomy to the United States in 1851.[15]

Episiotomy was advocated more and more in the early 1900s.[8,58] Leaders of the obstetrical community, especially Pomeroy (1918) and DeLee (1920), wrote papers advocating its frequent use.[29,60] Although it was not immediately accepted by practitioners, these papers began to change the climate of opinion toward the procedure. As late as 1915, a mail survey of prominent obstetricians indicated that few physicians utilized episiotomy on a routine basis.[66] However, in 1938 Diethelm reflected the opinion of the obstetrical community in asserting that the "indications (for episiotomy) are definitely established and need no defense."[30] It is worth emphasizing that this statement was made in the absence of definitive evidence for benefits from widespread use of episiotomy.

Important factors in its acceptance were changes in maternal mortality and rises in infant deaths from birth injuries that occurred in the 1920s. Physicians responded by establishing hospital committees to investigate each maternal death, and hospitals instituted rigid regulations.[74] From 1936 to 1955 maternal mortality dropped dramatically, in part because of improved quality of care, although the introduction of antibiotics and various social and economic factors also had an effect. This drop in mortality fostered a faith in technology, including episiotomy, and encouraged the view that labor and delivery are abnormal processes which benefit from medical intervention.

After World War II, episiotomy was used with increasing frequency. In 1915, it was done in less than 5% of all vaginal deliveries[66] whereas in 1979, 64.2% of vaginal deliveries had episiotomies.[55] Unfortunately, the percentage of episiotomies done in primigravidas is not known, although it is known to be higher in this group than with subsequent deliveries. Estimates of episiotomy rates in primigravidas range from 50% to 90%.[26,28,31,50,76] Large university-affiliated medical centers often have rates above 90% in primigravidas, indicating routine use. The rate in multigravidas is estimated to be 25% to 30%.

The rise in the rate of episiotomy in the United States has been paralleled by increases in other countries. The national rate of episiotomy was 21% in Great Britain in 1958 and rose to as much as 91% in some hospitals in 1978.[16] However, the overall rate of episiotomy is lower in most countries than it is in the United States. Episiotomies are down in 8% of deliveries in the Netherlands, where over 40% of women deliver their babies at home.[32] It is also worth noting that the episiotomy rate in home delivery in the United States is reported to be less than 10%.[50,52]

The recent obstetrical literature contains almost no comment on the efficacy and safety of episiotomy. Instead, reports focus on alternative techniques,[7,25,29,60] especially whether to use a mediolateral or midline approach. Obstetricians in the United States believe that the midline procedure is preferable, whereas in Great Britain the mediolateral approach is preferred.[16,31,61] Stated advantages of the median incision include easier repair, better healing, less postpartum pain and dyspareunia (pain during intercourse), and less blood loss. The mediolateral incision apparently has less risk of third-degree extension.[61]

A number of new techniques, including prepared childbirth classes, the Lamaze method, and Kegel's exercises to improve pelvic floor functioning[65] have helped women to become more involved in the birth process in recent years. Although benefits from these techniques are reported, such as fewer complications and less use of drugs for pain relief during labor,[44,69] the effects of these methods have not been adequately assessed.[40] They probably have affected the need for episiotomy and other interventions; however, one study that includes rates of episiotomy for Lamaze-prepared patients versus controls finds rates of 95% or greater in both groups, indicating that the use of childbirth preparation itself does not necessarily lower the rates of episiotomy. Still, these techniques probably have affected the rationale for episiotomy, which will be discussed in the next section.

Benefits of Episiotomy

Episiotomy is said to prevent third-degree lacerations,* pelvic relaxation, and damage to the fetal head while enabling a simpler repair of the incision. We will examine the data assessing these benefits.

Prevention of Lacerations

Prior to the advent of frequent episiotomies, the rates of laceration among primigravidas ranged from 10% to nearly 90%, and among multigravidas from less than 5% to just over 15%.[15,48] However, these early studies are difficult to interpret because of differences in definition of lacerations. If one focuses on series reported since 1920 and concerns oneself only with the rate of third-degree laceration, among women not having an episiotomy reported rates are 0% to 6.4% (Table 1). The rate of third-degree lacerations in series with episiotomy ranges in 23 separate reports from 0% to 23.9%.** The broad range of laceration rates makes comparisons in these studies complicated and no doubt reflects differences in definition as well as variations in patient populations and the skill of the accoucheur.

A few studies have compared the rate of laceration in patients who received episiotomy with those who did not (Table 2).[14,24,58] Although these studies were not randomized and control groups were not well matched for potential risk factors, they are of some interest. Child found a rate of third-degree laceration of 5.2% in 58 primigravidas who did not receive episiotomies, whereas 54 women who did have episiotomies had no third-degree lacerations.[24] Similarly, Nugent found that 2.3% of 130 women undergoing episiotomy had third-degree lacerations compared with 6.4% of the 72 women without episiotomy.[58] He reported that 9% of the 110 women who received mediolateral incisions and 13 of the 20 women who received midline incisions had extensions (tearing beyond the original incision). On

---

*Lacerations are also called tears, and in the context of an episiotomy will usually refer to a spontaneous extension of the incision. Third-degree laceration means a tear into the anus. Some authors describe a fourth-degree laceration as one extending into the rectum, but those with third-degree lacerations are included here.

**References are available from the authors.

Table 1
Percentage of women having an episiotomy
complicated by third-degree lacerations,
by type of incision, 33 studies, 1919-1980

Type	Number of Studies	Third-Degree Lacerations Range (Percent)	Weighted Average (Percent)
Episiotomy			
Midline	15	0.2 - 23.9	3.6
Mediolateral	6	0.0 - 9.0	0.6
Unspecified	5	0.0 - 17.2	4.0
No Episiotomy	7	0.0 - 6.4	2.0

the other hand, a small controlled series developed retrospectively also found increased numbers of third-degree lacerations among those receiving episiotomies.[14]

During the period from 1965 to 1973 in Cardiff, Wales, the incidence of episiotomy doubled from 24.4% to 46.7%, whereas the reported occurrence of lacerations decreased from 18.2% to 14.9%, despite a concomitant increase in the use of forceps from 6.4% to 16.6%.[20] Although this study suggests a possible decrease in lacerations related to the use of episiotomy, it is only a temporal association not a case of cause and effect.

Several birthing centers where episiotomy is not done routinely show rates of third-degree laceration of 0% to 3.6% and rates of first- and second-degree laceration requiring repair of 27% to 47%[66] (H. Maicki, G. Cranch, personal communications, 1980). The Farm, a rural Tennessee farming collective, reported that in 801 deliveries without episiotomy 4 (0.5%) had third-degree lacerations compared with 4.5% of 199 deliveries with episiotomies.[36] It was not clear whether or not the latter group included intentional third-degree incisions.

Several factors, including gravidity, breech presentation, use of forceps, and rapidity of the second stage of labor affect the rate of occurrence of perineal laceration.[31,48] In addition, the type of episiotomy (midline vs. mediolateral), the use and type of anesthesia, and the experience of the practitioner may be related to the occurrence of laceration.

Taken as a whole, the available data do not indicate that episiotomy offers a clear benefit to women in terms of decreased numbers of lacerations. There are certainly fewer reported lacerations today than there were in earlier years. However, third-degree lacerations occur in low frequency with and without episiotomy, and many factors, including healthier women, improved

Table 2
Comparison of laceration rates in women
with and without episiotomy, 3 studies, 1919 - 1979

Study	Number of Women	Number of Women with Third-Degree Lacerations
Child (1919)		
Episiotomy	54	0
Control	58	3
Nugent (1935)		
Episiotomy	130	3
Control	72	5
Brendsel (1979)		
Episiotomy	29	5
Control	29	0

obstetrical techniques, and better case selection could explain the reported decrease.

Prevention of Pelvic Relaxation

The prevention of long-term damage to the pelvic floor and interference with sexual function are frequently cited reasons for episiotomy, but few studies have tested this clinical hypothesis. An uncontrolled report of 240 primigravidas described 8 women with pelvic relaxation when examined 6 weeks after delivery.[30]

A study comparing 130 women who had received episiotomies and 72 controls who had not found normal pelvic support at 6 weeks in nearly 75% of the women with episiotomies but only 56% of the controls.[58] Serious pelvic relaxation was found in 1.5% of women with episiotomies and 9.7% of the controls. In the control group, increasing age and presumably increasing parity were associated with unsatisfactory results. A third study compared the results of labor and delivery in about 1000 clinic patients delivered by interns from 1920 to 1925, when women completed labor without episiotomy, to a similar number of women delivered between 1930 and 1934, when delivery included midline episiotomy and prophylactic low forceps.[2] Vaginal surgery and injury to the pelvic floor were greatly decreased in the episiotomy group. Although striking, the interpretation of these studies is complicated by the nonequivalence of study and control groups, a relatively small sample size, knowledge by the examiner as to assignment of women to study and control groups, and other serious methodological problems. In addition, the question of long-term status of pelvic relaxation was not addressed.

At the same time, a small study comparing 29 women giving birth with episiotomy with 29 matched controls giving birth without an episiotomy showed no statistically significant differences between the two groups in rates of pelvic relaxation as measured by perionometer readings and the occurrence of rectocele. There were 10 cases of vaginal numbness in the episiotomy group and only one in the control group. Although interesting, the report contains little detail and is hard to interpret.

The trend in the United States toward reduced family size may indicate a decreased need to protect the pelvic floor, since the anatomical structures are stressed less frequently.[54,71,72] On the other hand, pelvic relaxation may not reflect a cumulative effect, and a single severe stress may induce maximum damage. Data are not yet available to assess this effect on the pelvic floor.

In summary, the role of episiotomy in preventing serious pelvic relaxation has not been adequately studied. Indeed, the presence of pelvic relaxation may be further affected by cultural practices that lead to poor development of the pelvic floor, in particular the pubococcygeal muscles.[65] The section on risk gives some data on sexual functioning after episiotomy. Several other studies are underway that may shed light on the problem.

Prevention of Damage to the Newborn Baby:
Shortening the Second Stage of Labor

Fetal asphyxia and increased trauma to the head are thought to cause cerebral palsy and mental retardation, but few data exist to support the utilization of episiotomy to prevent brain damage to the fetus.[61] Indeed, studies of cerebral palsy and mental retardation suggest that the large majority of factors which produce such problems occur prior to labor and delivery.[1]

Episiotomy is one of several techniques used in obstetrics to shorten the second stage of labor,[51] a practice of unproved benefit to the fetus.[12,19,27,77] In one study, 22 women with uncomplicated pregnancies were randomly allocated into fast- and slow-delivery groups.[77] The fast-delivery process included early episiotomy, encouragement of pushing, and the use of forceps in case of delay. The authors concluded that benefit was found in faster delivery, but small sample size precluded accurate assessment of all the factors that were included in the study. Moreover, the outcome measures that seem of greatest interest, the scalp blood pH and Apgar score, were not significantly different in the two groups.

Slow distention of the pelvic tissues is less traumatic than sudden or rapid stretching and results in fewer lacerations and less need for episiotomy.[7,52] Caldeyro-Barcia has described a study in progress in 20 medical centers in Latin America that related to the subject of speeding labor and delivery.[18] If the membranes are artificially ruptured, the labor is shortened by 30 to 40 minutes. However, the cranial bones are misaligned in 50% of early rupture cases and in 34% of late rupture cases, apparently because of the lack of amniotic fluid and the intensity of contractions. Such changes have been shown to be associated with cerebral damage and abnormal electroencepholographic examinations.

The National Institutes of Health (NIH) has supported two studies relating the time of labor to the outcome of delivery, both as part of the Collaborative Study of Cerebral Palsy, Mental Retardation and Other Neurological and Sensory Disorders of Infancy and Childhood.[35,56] Friedman and co-workers examined correlates of abnormal mental and motor examinations in 1,194 infants at 8 and 12 months of age and found no particular correlation between clinical labor diagnosis and infant normality.[35] In the other study, Nelson and Broman studied 50 children with severe neurological abnormalities in comparison with a large control group and reported no difference between the handicapped group and the control group in mean duration of the first or second stage of labor.[56] Another large perinatal study in Great Britain that included over 17,000 live births demonstrated no differences related to the duration of the second stage in outcomes among term infants without fetal distress.[17] It is important to recognize in this and the NIH studies that artificially accelerated labors were not distinguished from labors shortened by other factors (e.g., multiparity). Hence, although one can comment on the length of labor, the issue of medical intervention is not specifically addressed in these reports.

The frequent use of oxytocics, pain-killing drugs, and epidural anesthesia and other practices related to shortening the second stage are associated with some risk to mother and baby.[63] In addition, the enhanced contractions threaten the fetus, so it is argued that electronic fetal monitoring must be used, a procedure with its own attendant risks.[3,63] The loss of maternal control over the birth process that is inherent in the use of anesthetics limits the participation of women in the control of delivery, a factor which may affect rates of laceration and pelvic relaxation.[40,41] At the same time, the standard use of the lithotomy position in hospital deliveries not only has detrimental physiological effects but also mechanically stresses the perineum, thereby decreasing the natural distensibility of the perineal tissues and probably increasing the risk of laceration.[10,40,61]

These studies suggest no clear benefit for shortening the second stage of labor. Indeed, speeding the second stage by active pushing could be harmful to the fetus and almost certainly leads to increased episiotomies and perhaps lacerations.

Summary

Although studies are lacking, clinical experience indicates that there are some cases, such as when the fetus is large and labor is prolonged, where episiotomy may be indicated. This, however, does not necessarily mean that routine episiotomy can be justified. It is incumbent on those advocating a procedure to prove benefit in adequately designed clinical trials. In the case of episiotomy, no published studies adequately quantify the real benefits of the procedure.

Risks of Episiotomy

Episiotomy can be complicated by extension of the incision (see earlier), unsatisfactory anatomical results,[6,26] increased blood loss,[26,28,57] dyspareunia,[8,16,26] postpartum pain, and infection.[30,37] Relatively rare problems include endometriosis in the episiotomy scar and nonhealing of the episiotomy.[30,42] Yet no published study specifically addresses the risks or side effects of episiotomy, and the importance of these complications can at best be inferred from data collected for another purpose, often not considering potentially confounding factors such as the type of anesthesia or treatment after delivery.

Pain and Edema

Pain following episiotomy appears to be almost universal. Yet, rates of moderate to severe pain are only found in studies of pain medication or different episiotomy techniques and range from less than 1% to as high as 60%, with 15% to 25% having continued pain after 3 days.[4,11] Bloomfield and Hurwitz note that moderate to severe pain is common among postepisiotomy patients and state that these otherwise normal women are ideal subjects for clinical trials of medication for pain and inflammation.[9] In over 30 reports, common medications (e.g., codeine, aspirin, and propoxyphene) as well as proteolytic enzymes (e.g., chymotrypsin) have been tested.*

*References available from authors.

Rarely is consideration given to potential confounding factors such as type of anesthesia, suturing material, patient anxiety, or the hypoestrogenic effects of postpartum breastfeeding.[16,34,64] A randomized controlled clinical trial of two methods of mediolateral episiotomy repair reported perineal pain requiring analgesia in 85% of primigravidas.[16] Edema also occurs immediately following episiotomy and may persist beyond 3 days.[4,11] Reported rates vary from about 10% to about 45% on the first day following delivery.

Dyspareunia (pain during intercourse) is rarely mentioned in the obstetrical literature as a complication of episiotomy.[8,16] Among 237 women seen 3 months postpartum, approximately one-half attempted intercourse in the first 6 weeks, and nearly two thirds reported pain or discomfort.[6] At 3 months, 56 women (23%) reported persistent dyspareunia, a finding inversely related to parity. Fifteen of these women reported the pain as severe. In another study, dyspareunia was reported in 85% of primigravidas within 4 weeks of delivery; 45% continued to report painful intercourse more than 4 weeks postpartum.[16]

Two recent British studies about episiotomy pain warrant special mention. Among 1,795 women who had attended prenatal classes, those with episiotomy were more likely to experience perineal pain a week after delivery than women with lacerations (37% vs. 15%).[47] Women who had episiotomy reported increased dyspareunia relative to women with lacerations. Almost 19% of women who underwent episiotomy experienced dyspareunia for more than 3 months compared with 11% who had lacerations. In a second report, 101 primigravidas were interviewed within 24 hours of delivery and sent a questionnaire by mail 3 months later.[62] Nearly one-third of the 69 women who responded to the mail survey reported a problem requiring medical attention, 15% reported episiotomy-related pain at 3 months postpartum, and about three fourths related dyspareunia to episiotomy. Labor pain did not correlate with episiotomy pain, whereas attendance at prenatal classes decreased the use of pain medications. It should be kept in mind that episiotomies done in the United Kingdom are usually mediolateral.

Infection

Infections associated with episiotomy include febrile morbidity, stitch abscesses (approximately 1%), and wound infections (0.5% to 3.0%).[26,30,33,37] Because reported studies were not controlled, nor were there comparisons with women who suffered morbidity without episiotomy, firm conclusions are impossible to draw. In addition, the rates of infection with laceration are not known.

Death from infection secondary to episiotomy is rarely considered. Yet Shy reported three deaths in Seattle between 1969 and 1977 from this cause, accounting for 20% of the maternal mortality in King County.[70] Two patients had necrotizing fasciitis, and one had clostridial myonecrosis (gas gangrene). Likewise, Ewing and colleagues studied 49,007 births in Kern County, California, between 1969 and 1976.[33] There were 11 maternal deaths, 3 of which were due to infection related to episiotomy. Another report of 4 cases of postpartum necrotizing fasciitis indicated that all 3 women undergoing vaginal delivery had an episiotomy, although no relationship was drawn between illness and the procedure.[38] Although uncommon, this severe complication could account for a substantial percentage of maternal deaths nationwide.

In summary, although rarely associated with a life-threatening problem, episiotomy can be a source of serious morbidity to young mothers who already have major personal and social adjustments to undergo.

Discussion

As one of the fundamental processes of human life, birth is clearly not merely a medical issue. Historically, it has been surrounded by cultural taboos, beliefs, and rituals. Recent feminist literature emphasizes the control of the birth process by men as a key part of our cultural background.[10,41,67] Obstetrics has been used, this literature states, as a method of social control.[67] Whereas such formulations are an important part of the women's health movement and are certainly related to the theme of this paper, interest here focuses on the lack of scientific data to support the widespread use of episiotomy. Unquestioning faith in technology, the dramatic benefits of obstetrics to some, and the development of the technological capability to do procedures such as episiotomy with an apparent minimum of risk have all played a role in fostering such widespread use.

Others have observed that technologies of unquestioned benefit for particular groups of people tend to get used for wider and wider indications.[63] The end result is that people with little or no need for the technology have it applied to their condition. This seems to be a particular problem in obstetrics, where complicated and uncomplicated cases are side by side, and where the uncomplicated can quickly become complicated.

We do not doubt the need for episiotomy in some cases, although even these indications have not been well studied. We do see episiotomy as a classical example of overutilization. In such a complex area, few have taken a balanced position. Moore is an exception: ''The absence of stitches during the lying-in period is a great advantage from every point of view...If a second-degree tear seems inevitable despite all precautions, it is preferable to do an episiotomy."[52]

This leaves the question of the appropriate rate of episiotomy. Midwives generally attempt to avoid episiotomy, as do practitioners in the recently established birthing centers. The data identified in this chapter indicate that rates of episiotomy vary in birthing centers from around 19% where the midwife is the primary provider to 39% where obstetricians are more dominant. We would therefore estimate that one episiotomy in every five deliveries is a reasonable minimum. Such a minimum is only an average and would, for example, be higher in primigravidas.

The scientific literature on episiotomy is sadly deficient. One would have hoped to find randomized controlled clinical trials testing proposed benefits. However, other research would have been useful. Chalmers and Richards proposed that trials of techniques such as episiotomy should include groups in which there is no planned intervention except continuous emotional support.[21] Little is known about the rates of long-term pelvic relaxation, even without episiotomy. For example, does pelvic relaxation tend to persist or does it improve with time or with exercise? A study to document in quantitative terms the extent and nature of pain and infection in women undergoing episiotomy and in properly selected controls might help change the attitude that episiotomy is a procedure without risks.

Data to support the widespread use of episiotomy are not available. In addition, obstetricians have largely ignored the demonstrable risks of episiotomy. In particular, the occurrence of pain that can persist for months after delivery bolsters the argument that episiotomy should be used judiciously. We doubt that women would agree to have routine episiotomies if they were fully informed as to the evidence for benefit, along with the expected rates of pain and infection. The absence of evidence of benefit makes it even more imperative than usual that women be informed and given the opportunity to make a choice for themselves.

REFERENCES

1. Alberman E. Facts and figures. In Chard T, Richards M (eds): *Benefits and hazards of the new obstetrics.* Philadelphia, JB Lippincott Co, 1977.

2. Aldridge AH, Wootson P. Analysis of end-results of labor in primiparas after spontaneous versus prophylactic methods of delivery. *J Obstet Gynecol* 30:554–565, 1935.

3. Banta HD, Thacker SB. Assessing the costs and benefits of electronic fetal monitoring. *Obstet Gynecol Surv* 35:627–642, 1979.

4. Bare WW, Fine ES. Prophylaxis of episiotomy pain: A controlled study of oral trypsins on the postpartum course. *Am J Obstet Gynecol* 87:268–271, 1963.

5. Barker-Benfield GJ. *The horrors of the half-known life*. New York, Harper Colophon Books, 1976.

6. Beischer NA. The anatomical and functional results of mediolateral episiotomy. *Med J Aust* 2:189–195, 1967.

7. Beynon CL. The normal second stage of labour. *J Obstet Gynaecol Br Emp* 64:815–820, 1957.

8. Beynon CL. Midline episiotomy as a routine procedure. *J Obstet Gyneacol Br Common* 81:126–130, 1974.

9. Bloomfield SS, Hurwitz HN. Tourniquet and episiotomy pain as test models for aspirin-like analgesics. *J Clin Pharmacol* 10:361–369, 1970.

10. Boston Women's Health Book Collective. *Our bodies, ourselves*. New York, Simon & Schuster, 1976.

11. Boutselis JG, Sollars RJ. The effect of proteolytic enzymes on episiotomy pain and swelling. *Ohio State Med J* 60:551–553, 1964.

12. Bowe NL. Intact perineum: A slow delivery of the head does not adversely affect the outcome of the newborn. *J Nurse-Midwifery* 26:5–11, 1981.

13. Bowes WA Jr. *Obstetrical medication and infant outcome: A review of the literature*. The effects of obstetrical medication on fetus and infant (Monograph). Monographs of the Society for Research in Child Development Serial no.137, 35:3–23, 1970.

14. Brendsel C, Peterson G, Mehl LE. Episiotomy: Facts, fictions, figures, and alternatives. In Stewart L and Stewart D (eds). *Compulsory hospitalization or freedom of choice in childbirth?* (Vol I) Marble Hill, MO, National Association of Parents and Professionals for Safe Alternatives in Childbirth, 1979.

15. Broomall AE. The operation of episiotomy as a prevention of perineal ruptures during labor. *Am J Obstet Dis Women Child* 11:517–527, 1878.

16. Buchan PC, Nicholls JAJ. Pain after episiotomy—a comparison of two methods of repair. *J Roy Coll Gen Pract* 30:297–300, 1980.

17. Butler NR., Alberman ED, (eds). *Perinatal problems*. London, Livingstone, 1960.

18. Caldeyro-Barcia R. Some consequences of obstetrical interference. *Birth Fam J* 2:34–38, 1977.

19. Caldeyro-Barcia R. The influence of maternal bearing-down efforts during second stage on fetal well-being. *Birth Fam J* 6:17–21, 1979.

20. Chalmers I, Zlosnik JE, Johns KA, et al. Obstetric practice and outcome of pregnancy in Cardiff residents. *Br Med J* 1:735–738, 1976.

21. Chalmers I, Richards M. Intervention and causal inference in obstetric practice. In Chard T, Richards M (eds). *Benefits and hazards of the new obstetrics*. Philadelphia, JB Lippincott Co, 1977.

22. Chalmers I. Implications of the current debate on obstetric practice. In Kitzinger S, Davis JA (eds). *The place of birth*. New York, Oxford University Press, 1978.

23. Chang NK, Chang CF. Median episiotomy. *West J Surg* 51:7–9, 1943.

24. Child CG Jr.: Episiotomy: Its relation to the proper conduct of the perineal stage of labor. *Med Rec* 96:142–144, 1919.

25. Coats PM, Chan KK, Wilkins M, et al. A comparison between midline and mediolateral episiotomies. *Br J Obstet Gynaecol* 87:408–412, 1980.

26. Cogan R, Edmonds EP. The unkindest cut? *Contemp Obstet Gynecol* 9:55–59, 1977.

27. Cohen WR. Influence of the duration of second stage labor on perinatal outcome and puerperal morbidity. *Obstet Gynecol* 49:266–269, 1977.

28. Conn LC, Vant JR, Cantor MM. A critical analysis of blood loss in 2000 obstetric cases. *Am J Obstet Gynecol* 42:768–785, 1941.

29. DeLee JB. The prophylactic forceps operation. *Am J Obstet Gynecol* 1:34–44, 1920.

30. Diethelm MW. Episiotomy; technique of repair. *Ohio Med J* 34:1107–1110, 1938.

31. Douglas RG, Stromme WB. Operative obstetrics. In *Management of delivery trauma*. (3rd ed) New York, Appleton-Century-Crofts, 1976.

32. Ettner FM: Study of obstetrics: 1975; with data and details of a working physicians' home OB service. In Stewart L, Stewart D (eds). *Safe alternatives in childbirth* (Vol 1) Chapel Hill, MO, National Association of Parents and Professionals for Safe Alternatives in Childbirth, 1976.

33. Ewing TL, Smale LE, Elliott FA. Maternal deaths associated with postpartum vulvar edema. *Am J Obstet Gynecol* 134:173–179, 1979.

34. Falicov CJ. Sexual adjustment during first pregnancy and postpartum. *Am J Obstet Gynecol* 117:991–1000, 1973.

35. Friedman EA, Niswander KR, Sachtlebel MR. Dysfunctional labor. XI. Neurologic and developmental effects on surviving infants. *J Obstet Gynecol* 33:785–791, 1969.

36. Gaskin IM. Community alternatives to high technology birth. In Holmes HB, Hoskins BB, Gross M (eds). *Birth control and controlling birth.* Clifton, NJ, Humana Press Inc, 1980.

37. Giglio FA, Germany WW, Roberts P. The infected episiotomy. *Obstet Gynecol* 25:502–508, 1965.

38. Golde S, Ledger WJ. Necrotizing fasciitis in postpartum patients. *Obstet Gynecol* 150:670–673, 1977.

39. Gusman H. The prophylactic use of episiotomy in primipara. *Ohio State Med J* 28:653–656, 1932.

40. Hahn SR, Paige KE. American birth practices: A critical review. In Parsons J (ed). *Psychobiology of sex differences and sex roles.* New York, Hemisphere Publications, 1980.

41. Haire D. *The cultural warping of childbirth.* A Special Report. Hillside, NJ, International Childbirth Education Association, 1972.

42. Hambrick E, Abcarian H, Smith D. Perineal endometrioma in episiotomy incisions: Clinical features and management. *Dis Colon Rect* 22:550–555, 1979.

43. Hiatt HH. Protecting the medical commons: Who is responsible? *N Engl J Med* 293:235–241, 1975.

44. Hughey MJ, McElin TW, Young T. Maternal and fetal outcome of Lamaze-prepared patients. *Obstet Gynecol* 51:643–647, 1978.

45. Kaltreider DF, Dixon DM. A study of 710 complete lacerations following central episiotomy. *South Med J* 41:814–820, 1948.

46. Kantor HI, Rember R, Tabio P, et al. Value of shaving the pudendal-perineal area in delivery preparation. *Obstet Gynecol* 25:509–512, 1965.

47. Kitzinger S, Walters R. *Some women's experiences of episiotomy.* London, National Childbirth Trust, 1981.

48. Manton WP. A plea for episiotomy. *Am J Obstet Dis Women Child* 18:226–235, 1885.

49. Marieskind HI. An evaluation of caesarean section in the United States. US Department of Health, Education, and Welfare, June, 1979.

50. Mehl LE. Research on alternatives in childbirth: What can it tell us about hospital practice? In Stewart L, Stewart D (eds). *21st century obstetrics now!* Marble Hill, MO, National Association of Parents and Professionals for Safe Alternatives in Childbirth, 1977.

51. Mehl LE. The outcome of home delivery research in the United States. In Kitzinger S, Davis JA (eds). *The place of birth.* New York, Oxford University Press, 1978.

52. Moore WMO. The conduct of the second stage. In Chard T, Richards M (eds). *Benefits and hazards of the new obstetrics.* Philadelphia, JB Lippincott Co, 1977.

53. Murray RR. Operative intervention in normal labor and delivery. *Obstet Gynecol Ann* 9:195–212, 1980.

54. National Center for Health Statistics/National Center for Health Services Research. *Health United States,* 1978, Hyattsville, Md, HEW Publication no. (PHS) 78–1232. Dec 1978.

55. National Center for Health Statistics. *Data from the Hospital Discharge Survey.* Furnished by Eileen McCarthy, Feb 1981.

56. Nelson KB, Broman SH. Perinatal risk factors in children with serious motor and mental handicaps. *Ann Neurol* 2(5):371–377, 1977.

57. Newton M, Mosey LM, Egli GE, et al. Blood loss during and immediately after delivery. *Obstet Gynecol* 17:9–18, 1961.

58. Nugent FB. The primiparous perineum after forceps delivery. *Am J Obstet Gynecol* 30:249–256, 1935.

59. Ould F. *Treatise of midwifery*. Dublin, Nelson and Connor, 1742, p 145.

60. Pomeroy RH: Shall we cut and reconstruct the perineum for every primipara? *Am J Obstet Dis Women Child* 78:211–220, 1918.

61. Pritchard JA, MacDonald PC. *Williams Obstetrics*. (16th ed) New York, Appleton-Century-Crofts, 1980.

62. Reading AE, Sledmere CM, Cox DN, et al. How women view post-episiotomy pain. *Br Med J* 284:243–246, 1982.

63. Richards MPM. A place of safety? An examination of the risks of hospital delivery. In Kitzinger S, Davis JA (eds). *The place of birth*. New York, Oxford University Press, 1978.

64. Richardson AC, Lyon JB, Graham EE, et al. Decreasing postpartum sexual abstinence time. *Am J Obstet Gynecol* 126:416–417, 1976.

65. Rodway HE. A statistical study on the effect of exercise on childbearing. *J Obstet Gynaecol Br Emp* 54:77–85, 1947.

66. Rothschild CJ. Episiotomy, a perineal safety measure. *J Indiana Med Soc* 8:416–418, 1915.

67. Ruzek SB. *The women's health movement*. New York, Praeger Publishers, 1978.

68. Schmidt J. The first year at Stanford University's family birth room. *Birth Fam J* 7:169–174, 1980.

69. Scott JR, Rose NB. Effect of psychoprophylaxis (Lamaze preparation) on labor and delivery in primiparas. *N Engl J Med* 294:1205–1207, 1976.

70. Shy KK, Eschenbach DA. Fatal perineal cellulitis from an episiotomy site. *Obstet Gynecol* 54:292–298, 1979.

71. US Bureau of the Census. *Historical statistics of the United States, colonial times to 1970*. Washington DC, 1975.

72. US Bureau of the Census. Fertility of American women, June, 1979. *Curr Pop Rep* 1980; series P-2-350.

73. Wendt WP, Wolfgram R. Episirectomy. *Obstet Gynecol* 18:626–629, 1961.

74. Wertz RW, Wertz DC. *Lying-in, a history of childbirth in America*. New York, The Free Press, 1977.

75. Wertz DC. Man-midwifery and the rise of technology. In Holmes HB, Hoskins BB, Gross M (eds). *Birth control and controlling birth*. Clifton, NJ, Humana Press Inc, 1980.

76. Willmott J. Too many episiotomies. *Midwives Chron Nurs Notes* 93:46–49, 1980.

77. Wood C, Ng KH, Hounslow D, et al. Time—an important variable in normal delivery. *J Obstet Gynaecol Br Commonw* 80:295–300, 1973.

SUBMITTED: APRIL, 1981
REVISED & ACCEPTED: MARCH, 1982

CESAREAN SECTION

Helen I. Marieskind

Cesarean section is a surgical procedure in which the fetus is removed from the mother by an incision made through her abdominal and uterine walls. There are several types of cesarean surgery presently in use in the United States, and these procedures are described in this chapter. Also included is a historical perspective on cesarean surgery, characteristics of the cesarean population, a discussion of complications, possible explanations for the recent rise in cesareans, and educational activities for expectant parents.

Types of Cesarean Procedures

Cesarean procedures are classified as either primary (the first cesarean) or secondary (repeat cesareans with a subsequent pregnancy). They may be performed for absolute indications, meaning there is no other method by which a living child can be delivered, or for relative indications. These refer to conditions about which the practitioner has decided an abdominal delivery offers qualitatively better chances for the survival of mother and child.

Distinctions among cesarean surgeries are based on the types of incision used in the uterus itself. The most common method used in the United States is known as the "low cervical," which accounted for 87.1% of all cesareans performed in the 1974 PAS Study[1] and probably a large percentage of the 8.1% listed as "type unspecified." The procedure involves making a horizontal, crescent incision into the abdomen just above the pubic bone with a similar incision into the lower uterine segment. This incision is preferred for both physiological and cosmetic reasons, since the wound heals more strongly and will be largely obscured by the pubic hair line. A variation on this procedure utilizes a vertical abdominal incision with a horizontal lower uterine segment incision, thereby maximizing benefits inherent in each procedure of less blood loss.

Although widely used in the early twentieth century, the "classical" pro-

---

Much of this material has been drawn from *An Evaluation of Caesarean Section in the United States*. Washington, D.C., U.S. Government Printing Office, 1979.

179

cedure was utilized in only 4% of the PAS cesarean surgeries studied in 1974.[1] It involves making a vertical incision into the center of the upper segment of the uterus. Generally for this type of procedure a vertical incision about 5 inches in length will also be made into the abdomen. This technique is usually only employed today in cases where the fetus is lying in a transverse position, for placenta praevia, and for extreme emergencies when the speed of access afforded by this procedure is essential.

"Extraperitoneal" cesarean sections have the objective of protecting the peritoneal cavity from an already infected uterus. This technique is rarely used (only 0.1% were reported in the 1974 PAS data)[1] although advocates acclaim its potential for reducing morbidity. The "extraperitoneal" cesarean comprises a transverse incision into the abdomen with portions of the peritoneal membrane being sutured together to leave the uterus exposed and isolated from the general peritoneal cavity. Disagreement is reported concerning the advisability of performing repeat extraperitoneal sections.[2,3]

Other types of cesareans are rarely used and accounted for only 0.8% of the 1974 PAS survey.[1] They were classified as "obstetrical hysterotomy," "peritoneal exclusion," "transperitoneal not otherwise specified," and "vaginal" cesarean. The latter involves a vertical incision in the cervix to gain access to the uterus.

All the foregoing techniques of cesarean surgery are contemporary adaptations of an ancient surgical procedure.

History of Cesarean Section Practice

Contrary to popular belief, cesarean section appears not to be connected with the birth of Julius Caesar, who most probably was born vaginally. The term is generally believed to come from the Roman *lex regia*, which ordered that an abdominal section must be performed on a dead or dying pregnant woman in order to save her child for the state. The *lex regia* eventually became known as the *lex Caesaria*. Some authorities, however, believe this stipulation to save infants was only added by the Church in the Middle Ages.

As with the origins of the name for the surgery, the origins of the procedure are also unclear. The folklore, lay and scholarly writings of ancient Europeans, Africans, Egyptians, Greeks, Romans, and Indians indicate that the technique was probably known to them. The early Jews definitely knew of cesarean section, as the Mishnah considers the rights of twins so delivered and the Talmud, dating from 400 A.D. states that a woman need not observe the usual days of purification after abdominal delivery.

Nonetheless, there is general agreement among historians that the procedure was first performed upon dead women to provide a separate burial for their children and occasionally upon dying women when the baby still showed signs of life. Christianity gave a new meaning to intrauterine life, and the Catholic Church encouraged the use of cesareans to offer the souls of unborn infants the chance of salvation. The church councils of Cologne (1280), Langres (1404), and Sens (1514) made the surgery obligatory, as did the Venetian Republic in 1608. Sixteenth century obstetricians Röslin and Guillemeau cite cesareans being performed to save the baby, but there are no records demonstrating that babies actually were saved.

Eventually cesarean section was used to assist living women, although frequently without success for either mother or baby. The mortality from this procedure became so excessive that from the sixteenth to the nineteenth centuries there was much opposition to its use. Craniotomy (puncturing the skull to collapse the head of the fetus so it can be removed) was preferred.

The most important advance in cesarean surgery came with the work of Adolf Kehrer and Max Sänger, who in 1882 discovered how to close the wound of the uterus with silk sutures, reputedly with an 80% success rate. Mortality dropped, and cesareans became more common.[4-7]

Opinions vary as to the date of the first cesarean section in the United States. One plausible record, although the exact dates differ, concerns a Dr. Jesse Bennett who operated upon his wife. After a desultory labor, Mrs. Bennett was faced with a choice of cesarean and the assurance she would most probably die, or craniotomy and the death of her baby. Electing the former, Dr. Bennett performed the surgery, either in 1794 or 1801. Mrs. Bennett reputedly survived for 37 more years, and the child lived until 77 years of age.[6]

At least equally as plausible is the attribution of the first cesarean in the United States to Francois Marie Prévost (1771–1842), a Louisiana physician who learned the technique in Paris. Prévost came to Louisiana in the early nineteenth century and encountered many malnourished, rickets-ridden slave women who suffered arduous labors and frequently died.

After reputedly saving both mother and child with his first cesarean procedure, Prévost performed the surgery on many others. He presumably trained other physicians, and records exist of 79 cesareans being performed between 1822 and 1877. Of these, 15 were performed in Louisiana between 1822 and 1861, resulting in 11 living mothers and 8 living children. Duffy notes the significance of the use of cesareans on slave women; the experimental nature and high mortality dissuaded physicians from risking white women's lives.[8]

Toward the close of the 1800's, the cesarean section was no longer a rarity.

Records are scarce, but those of the Charity Hospital in Shreveport, Louisiana, for example, show a cesarean rate of 1.3% between January 1, 1916, and June 30, 1918, with a maternal death rate of 30%.[9] Californian records from 1908 to 1933 showed a section rate of 3.1%, with 9 deaths in 290 cesareans.[10]

The shift to hospital births increased the survival rates for mothers and babies experiencing cesarean deliveries, although some sections were still performed in the home. A 1934 study of 56,000 home births in Iowa listed 111 home cesareans.[11]

The Papal Encyclical of 1930 *Casti Connubi* fostered the use of cesareans by forbidding the taking of an infant life to save a mother's. However, when no saving of infant life was demonstrated, the practice was decried at the 1933 White House Conference on Child Health and Protection, Fetal, Newborn and Maternal Mortality and Morbidity.[9]

The development of antibiotics, bloodbanks, improved surgical techniques, and improved training had all combined to increase the acceptability of cesarean surgery as an alternative to high- and mid-forceps used by the mid-1950s and 1960s. Cesarean section, a practice once used sparingly in only 3% to 5% of the deliveries nationwide, is now used in the births of 15% to 17% of the nation's babies. What was once extreme emergency surgery has, in the late 1970s and 1980s in the United States, become a standard accepted procedure annually used on approximately one in every 6 women giving birth (Table I).

Characteristics of the Cesarean Population

Women of all ages, parities (the number of pregnancies), races, educational and income levels, and marital states receive cesareans. The surgery is the third most common procedure for women aged 15 to 44 years, with a rate per 1,000 of 10.2 in 1978.[12]

From 1978 data (the most recent detailed analysis available), however, some women appear more at risk of cesareans than do others. Placek and Taffel note that women aged 30 years and over had about a 20% chance of delivering their babies by cesarean section as opposed to a range of 11.8% for those under 20 years to 16.4% for those aged 25 to 29 years.[13]

Women who have had one cesarean delivery are the most likely to have another. The 1974 analysis of the PAS data showed that 30% of cesareans performed (the largest category) were on women who had had a previous section.[1]

TABLE I

Cesarean Sections As a Percentage of All Deliveries, United States, 1968 to 1980*

Year	Number of Cesarean Sections (000)	Number of Deliveries (000)	Cesarean Sections (%)	Change in Number of Cesarean Sections(%)	Change in Number of Deliveries(%)
1968	172	3346	5.1		
*1970	195	3545	5.5	+ 7.8	+ 5.9
1971	194	3337	5.8	+ 5.5	− 5.9
1972	227	3224	7.0	+20.7	− 3.4
1973	246	3093	8.0	+14.3	− 4.1
1974	286	3122	9.2	+15.0	+ 0.9
1975	328	3048	10.8	+17.4	− 2.3
1976	378	3126	12.1	+12.0	+ 2.6
1977	455	3331	13.7	+13.2	+ 6.6
1978	510	3361	15.2	+10.9	+ 0.9
1979	599	3646	16.4	+ 7.9	+ 8.4
1980	619	3762	16.5	+ 0.6	+ 3.2

Based on data from National Center for Health Statistics; National Hospital Discharge Survey, 1968-1980, Washington, D.C., 1982.

*Data for 1969 are unavailable because the data collection system was altered.

Adapted from Marieskind, H.I. Women in the Health System - Patients, Providers, and Programs. St. Louis, The C.V. Mosby Co, 1980.

Primiparous women (women having their first delivery), particularly if they are over 30 years old, are also more likely to have cesareans. Primiparas experience a higher incidence of conditions that can warrant a cesarean, such as cephalopelvic disproportion, hemorrhage, dysfunctional labor, or pre-eclampsia.[14,15] Data from New York[16] and California[17] confirm these findings.

Grand multiparous women (six or more deliveries) are more likely to have cesareans than are women of 2 to 5 parities.[18,19] Performing cesarean sections on very young women who will have subsequent births may in time change these data, however. The 1972 National Natality Survey (the most recent) found that of those women with first legitimate live hospital births, 8.7% were sectioned, 6.3% of those with second births, 6.4% of third births, 5.7% of fourth births, but with the fifth or more birth 7.1% were by cesarean.[20]

Prior reproductive loss is associated with a higher incidence of cesarean section.[21] The 1972 Natality Survey confirms this, showing that 6.8% of women with no previous fetal loss had a cesarean, compared with 9.5% of those with one loss and 11.6% of those with two or more losses.[20]

Data on race of women who receive cesareans are complicated by the omission of racial data in a large percentage of deliveries. Bearing this in mind, data from 1970 through 1978 do show that the highest rate of cesareans occurred among white women in 1972, 1977, and 1978, among women of all other races in 1971, 1973, 1974, 1975, and 1976, and among women with no race stated in 1970. Overall there was not a substantial variation in cesarean rates by race of mother.[13] Other studies from 1951 to 1952,[14] the 1960s[22] and 1960 through 1975[17] have made similar findings.

Educational level may affect cesarean rates, since the 1972 National Natality Survey found a higher incidence in women who were college graduates.[20] Higher educational levels may also affect the amount of prenatal care sought which, in turn, may affect the incidence of cesareans, as discussed below.

Women who are private patients appear to have higher cesarean rates than do other women[18,20,23] although more recent data from Baltimore showed disproportionately high numbers of both groups having cesareans in different hospitals.[24] Women on public insurance programs such as Medicaid also have higher rates as do women with comprehensive insurance coverage.[20]

According to Placek and Taffel, married women were also more likely to deliver by cesarean section, although the difference is small—15.5% for married women compared with 13.3% for those unmarried. The high percentage of cesareans—18.1%—among those whose marital status was not stated may invalidate these findings, however.[13]

A woman's residence may affect the likelihood of her undergoing surgical birth. The 1972 National Natality Survey,[20] a New York City study,[18] and a Swedish study[25] all showed a higher incidence among women residing in metropolitan areas. These data may be biased due to the practice of referring complicated cases to large tertiary centers, which are usually located in metropolitan areas.

The relationship of cesarean section to prenatal care is less clear. In Petitti's 1960–1975 California study, less prenatal care was associated with a lower cesarean incidence.[17] The 1972 national data show that the highest cesarean rates occurred among women who had no prenatal care (7.3%) and women who had the greatest number of visits, 20 or more, to a physician (16.6%).[20] Petitti suggests three explanations for the relationship found in California: (1) that a higher cesarean incidence occurs because women who know they are high risk seek more and earlier care, (2) because of earlier detection of the fetus at risk, or (3) because of an increased emotional investment by the physician in the outcome of a pregnancy he or she has extensively monitored.[17]

Anticipated infant birth weight also affects cesarean incidence. Babies estimated to be 2,500 grams or less and/or of 36 weeks gestation or less, and those estimated to be 4,500 grams or more and/or 42 weeks gestation, are most likely to be delivered by cesarean.[14,16-18,20] Some studies show the most rapid increase in sections as having occurred with babies over 4,500 grams.[16,17]

Most women (42.6%) in the 1974 PAS Study used a combination of inhalation plus intravenous anesthesia, but anesthesia use varied by hospital size, region, and teaching status. Spinal anesthesia was also extensively used and was the second most commonly used method in teaching hospitals.[1] The 1972 National Natality Survey showed that of those women who received inhalation anesthesia, 7.8% gave birth by cesarean, whereas 15.5% of women who received spinal and epidural anesthesia had cesareans.[20]

The literature does cite use of local anesthesia for cesarean section[26,27] but this is not widely practiced as most physicians either are inexperienced with it or believed the dosage needed would be harmful to the fetus.

In 1974, 43.7% of women who had cesareans also experienced some other kind of surgery. The most common of these was tubal ligation performed on 16% of all cesarean patients, with other procedures bringing the total sterilization rate to 19.9%. Of these, 56.8% were performed on women between 15 and 29 years; they occurred most frequently in small hospitals in the South and West, and in nonteaching hospitals.[1]

In 1978 the highest rates of cesarean section were found in hospitals of 500 beds or more, 17.0 per 100 deliveries as compared with 10.1 in hospitals of fewer than 100 beds; and in proprietary hospitals (16.4) as opposed to voluntary nonprofit hospitals (15.8), and city, county, and state government hospitals (13.1).[13] The PAS data found that the highest rates were in teaching hospitals.[1] These findings are consistent with the referral of complicated obstetrical cases to tertiary centers, which are frequently large teaching hospitals.

In comparing cesarean incidence by region in 1978, the highest rates occurred in the Northeast, 17.6 per 100 deliveries, followed by the South (15.2), the West (14.6), and North Central (13.9). This order held true also in 1970.[13]

Length of hospital stay for a cesarean delivery in 1978 averaged nationally 6.7 days compared with 3.2 days for other deliveries. By region the mean lengths of stay were Northeast 7.5, North Central 7.0, South 6.3, and West

5.9 days.[13] The same regional order occurred for other deliveries with 3.8, 3.6, 3.0, and 2.4 days, respectively.

Nationally in 1978, of those women who had cesareans, 79.4% stayed in hospital 7 days or less, 18.6% stayed 8 to 14 days, and 2.0% stayed 15 days or more.

In summary, characteristics known to date about the cesarean population suggest that higher incidence is bimodally distributed: The oldest and youngest women, women with the least and the most education, women with the lowest and highest incomes, women with the lowest and highest parity, women with public insurance and the most comprehensive private plans, and women with the least and the most prenatal care.

The data further suggest the highest cesarean rates are found in the larger hospitals, in the Northeast, that women in the Northeast will stay in hospital longest, but that most women in the United States will stay 7 days or less.

Complications of Cesarean Section

Although the rise in cesarean sections is applauded by many professionals as providing improved outcome for infants, it is cause for concern for many others because of the costs—physical, financial, and psychological. Cesarean section is major surgery, with preliminary data from here and abroad suggesting a maternal mortality 2 to 26 times that of vaginal deliveries.[17,28-31] In addition, institutions generally report that at least one third of their cesarean patients have some postoperative infection.[32,33] Discomfort from abdominal and intestinal pain is reported by almost all patients, as is depression and exhaustion.

It is sometimes difficult with both the mother and the infant to distinguish between physical costs derived from the cesarean procedure per se and physical factors peculiar to the mother or infant for which the cesarean has been performed.

Shearer has summarized the various complications of cesarean section for the mother as follows:[34] Future cesarean deliveries;[35-40] psychological distress;[41] gas;[41] infection (intrauterine, cystitis, peritonitis, abscess, gangrene, generalized sepsis);[32,33,42,43] hemorrhage;[44] adhesions;[45] fistula;[46] sinuses;[47] wound dehiscence, subsequent uterine rupture;[48,49] injury to adjacent organs (e.g., uterus, bladder, bowel);[42] side effects of blood transfusion (e.g., hepatitis);[1] thromboemboli;[42,50] thrombophlebitis, aspiration pneumonia;[51,52] anesthesia accidents;[52] cardiac arrest;[1] cerebral vascular accidents;[1] and death.[1,53,54]

The principal physical cost to the infant born by cesarean is respiratory distress syndrome (RDS) or hyaline membrane disease (HMD).[55-57] This may be caused by iatrogenic prematurity[57] or when the baby is delivered before he or she is mature. The lungs of these infants lack pulmonary surfactant due to their prematurity, and hence the infant does not get sufficient oxygen to body tissues. Studies show elective deliveries to be a primary cause of RDS.[55,58]

If infants are allowed to initiate labor when they are ready, or if appropriate diagnostic testing is done to assess maturity prior to delivery,[59-61] much of the risk of RDS could be prevented.

Data on fetal mortality by mode of delivery are scarce and, again, it is often difficult to distinguish if mortality is from the cesarean per se or from conditions which lead to it. Data from PAS for 1974 and 1975 show that for the 212,000 single-birth, full-term hospital newborns delivered by cesarean, 732 died, which is a case fatality rate of 34 per 10,000. This contrasts with a case fatality of 12 per 10,000 for the 2,522 deaths among the 2,115,000 single-birth, full-term hospital newborns delivered other than by cesarean section in 1974 and 1975. Low birth weight plays a major role in infant mortality regardless of delivery mode, and most of the 1974 and 1975 infant deaths among those delivered by cesarean weighed less than 2,500 grams.[62]

Costs

Of equal concern are the rising financial costs associated with abdominal delivery. Costs of cesarean surgery are about three times those of vaginal delivery. With increased physician fees, supplies, and double the hospital stay, costs range today from $2,500 to $4,000. Cost calculations must also include the woman's loss of productivity due to the extended convalescence required following a cesarean and frequently the added expense of hiring household help to assist with household responsibilities such as other children and cleaning.[63] Intensive care costs for those infants born prematurely must also be included.

National health care costs could also be reduced by developing a more rational and individual policy toward repeat cesareans by allowing a trial of labor and vaginal deliveries for the estimated 50% of women for whom this is appropriate.[64] This shift in policy to individual evaluation from Cragin's 1916 dictum "once a Caesarean, always a Caesarean"[65] is now cautiously promoted by The American College of Obstetricians and Gynecologists[66] and could reduce the financial costs of cesarean section by more than 100 million dollars per year.[63]

Psychological Costs

Many women report feelings of inadequacy, guilt, regret, hostility toward the infant, and a sense of failure and helplessness in addition to fatigue, exhaustion, and malaise. Although it is unlikely that all these feelings are experienced by all women, to the degree that they exist, they are not constructive to maternal, and, ultimately, infant well-being.[41,67] Preventive measures are discussed below.

Reasons for the Rise in Cesareans

The rapid and continued increase in the cesarean section rate is the product of complex interrelated factors, and its study is hampered by a lack of valid data and scientific study.

Fear of Malpractice Suits

Two studies have reported on physician fear of a malpractice suit in the event of an adverse outcome if a cesarean had not been performed.[63,68] Studies of closed claims, however, show a high proportion of suits for alleged injury during a cesarean.[69] A few large settlements for failure to perform the surgery, however, are understandably conducive to being overly cautious and to order an operative delivery when there is any doubt.

Repeat Cesarean Policy

As noted under costs, until recently, the United States has had an almost universal policy of repeat cesarean surgery in subsequent pregnancies.[1] Although this is slowly changing, routine repeats continue to be the norm and, again, fear of malpractice suit in the event of an adverse outcome, especially when deviating from the norm, helps maintain repeat cesarean as an indication for one third of the cesareans performed annually.

Recent recommendations from the National Institute of Child Health and Human Development (NICHD) Consensus Conference[31] and The American College of Obstetricians and Gynecologists[66] will do much to erode this 64-year-old practice.[65] Recognizing the data from domestic studies such as those at the University of Texas, Robert B. Green Hospital,[64] and from such countries as England,[39] Jamaica,[37] and Ireland,[70] both bodies have recommended that with appropriate screening and management, women with a previous cesarean in whom the condition which warranted the surgery is no longer present, should be permitted a trial labor with the possibility of a vaginal delivery.

Obstetrical Training

Physician training today gives emphasis to surgical deliveries both through the literature and by practice. Training in normal obstetrics and low technology is rare, and studies of physicians and the literature have given several examples of little to no training in many areas, including auscultation by stethoscope, external cephalic version, vaginal breech deliveries, use of local anesthesia for cesareans, and clinical pelvimetry. By contrast, training in usage of electronic fetal monitoring, ultrasonic monitoring, and scalp sampling is extensive.[63,71] A recent finding in New York State that more cesareans are performed by younger rather than older obstetricians is consistent with this finding of the technological orientation of contemporary training.[72]

Belief in Superior Outcome from Cesarean Section

Throughout the United States, physician focus has shifted from the mother to the infant—to obtaining a perfect product. The literature frequently notes, and physicians confirm the belief, that the increased use of cesarean section, plus the widespread utilization of electronic fetal monitoring (EFM), are largely responsible for obtaining this improved product.[73] Declining infant and perinatal morbidity and mortality are cited as causal outcomes of the use of cesarean section and EFM. Increased use of cesarean delivery is said to be justified, therefore, in the interest of obtaining a superior outcome. That the rates have declined is true; that cesareans and EFM are responsible has not been proved. For example, a recent study shows that the greatest improvement in mortality is in the perinatal-neonatal rates in urban areas, which is also consistent with the availability of neonatal intensive care units in urban hospitals. There has also been great improvement in postneonatal mortality in rural areas. But the overall areas of fetal and neonatal rates are still two or three times higher with lower rates of decline than are the postneonatal rates.[74] Fetal and neonatal rates are those most subject to change through cesarean section, EFM, and as mentioned, neonatal intensive care units, yet they would not seem to be declining at a pace comparable with the increase in cesarean sections.

Three controlled trials, moreover, have shown no difference in outcome from use of EFM,[75-77] and with the exception of some conditions for which cesarean section has always been indicated, only circumstantial relationships have been established between cesarean section and birth outcome. Improved nutrition, prenatal care, availability of abortion, and decline in the congenital anomaly rate[78] may all be far more influential on outcome, and this has been analyzed by several authors. One community hospital, for example, noted in a 38-year review that its perinatal mortality had seen its major drop 2 years prior to a rapid increase in cesareans and to the introduction of EFM.[79] Other authors postulate that there may be an "all-or-nothing" aspect to fetal survival and that negative fetal outcomes are primarily determined by prebirth events.[80] Cesarean section and other obstetrical interventions would therefore have little effect.

Changing Indications for Cesarean Section

Changing indications are frequently cited as a reason for the increased cesarean rate.[42] As noted, indications may be absolute or relative, and the data suggest that the relative indications have not really changed, but rather more women are being identified as having "old" indications. Similarly, the question must be raised as to how much a climate accepting of cesarean sections, in and of itself, promotes more cesareans. One of the difficulties in evaluating this fifth factor in the rising rate is because there are no uniform definitions as to what constitutes an indication for a cesarean. When the data are examined by indication, most of the rise in cesareans comes from increased use of cesarean for cephalopelvic disproportion (CPD) or fetopelvic disproportion (FPD). This complication includes dystocia and also "failure to progress" or prolonged labor.[31] These terms are vague and nondiagnostic, yet are frequently given as the indication for cesarean. It is perhaps significant that these are conditions which cannot be evaluated after a delivery in the same way an EFM tracing can be assessed for signs of fetal distress which warranted intervention. Cephalopelvic disproportion, which was the indication for 28% of all PAS cesareans in 1974,[1] and is reported to have contributed to 25% to 30% of the increase in the cesarean rate from 1970 to 1978, appears to have become a "catch-all" diagnosis.[31]

The use of cesarean section for breech presentation has increased and is considered here under changing indications. Many institutions report that 60% to 90% of their breech presentations are delivered by cesarean. The data also suggest that belief in a superior outcome from cesarean breech delivery, as opposed to vaginal breech delivery, does seem warranted for very small or very large babies.[31] However, it is impossible to know if the seemingly superior outcome is due to the surgical intervention per se or the fact that cesarean breech data are being compared with data of vaginal breech deliveries managed by persons increasingly unskilled at such deliveries. Los Angeles County-University of Southern California, Women's Hospital completed a study demonstrating that with careful selection, term frank breeches were not associated with perinatal death. The authors noted that "although perinatal morbidity occurs with vaginal breech delivery, the significant maternal complications of elective C-section make C-section for term frank breech infants an unattractive policy."[81]

Age, Parity, and Fertility Characteristics

The sixth contributing factor concerns shifts in age, parity, and fertility characteristics of the childbearing population. Older women and primiparous women, both of whom have a higher risk of cesarean section, have increased in the childbearing population. The number of women over 30 years of age having their first babies and the number of primiparas have doubled from 1966 to 1980.[82]

Data from the National Center for Health Statistics also show that second babies are born at a 24- to 47-month interval after the previous birth. In 1974 there was a 5% increase since 1973 (the largest increase in a 10-year span) in the number of primiparas giving birth and a 16% increase over the previous year in the number of cesareans performed.[82] It is therefore to be expected, because of the policy of routine repeat surgery in the United States, that the cesarean rate would continue to exhibit an upward trend in 1976, 1977, and 1978 as those women, pregnant again, are sectioned and are joined by an increasing percentage of primiparous women who, in turn, receive cesareans.

Connected with this is the fact that the declining fertility rate and the average family size of two have led to the concept of "premium babies"— that "every baby counts." How much this concept is one expressed by parents and how much by obstetricians focusing on the fetus as patient is unclear. Belief that a cesarean section guarantees a perfect outcome would then justify surgical intervention to obtain this premium product.

Economics

The seventh factor concerns economic incentives, and although the data are consistent with the finding that an economic incentive contributes to the cesarean section rate, they do not definitively establish a causal relationship. Suggestions of an economic incentive should not be inferred as implying a deliberate calculation to do a cesarean to make money. Rather, a combination of economic factors can exert influence toward the more profitable, in this case surgical, approach, while at the same time providing no incentive to persist with a vaginal delivery. One source has noted a decline in the number of births per obstetrician from 260.7 in 1963 to 144.9 in 1976.[83] Despite declines in morbidity and mortality and improved prenatal care during this period, the rate for deliveries with complications has steadily increased from 19.4% in 1960 to 31.0% in 1978.[83](See Table 2.) During this period the salaries of obstetrician-gynecologists have also risen.[84]

Cesarean section may be attractive to the physician also because it involves a predictable expenditure of time. The added length of stay for cesarean deliveries is attractive to hospitals, particularly in light of the declining birthrate and empty obstetrical beds. Third party payment may also influence the decision to perform a cesarean section because the surgery is usually 100% covered, whereas vaginal deliveries are not completely covered. In addition, Medicaid reimburses from two thirds to double the amount that which is paid for vaginal deliveries. However, in prepaid plans where the economic incentive is to lower hospitalization, cesarean section rates have also risen. Much smaller increases have also been found in institutions relying heavily on midwives.[63]

Obstetrical Technology

It is extremely difficult to pinpoint the effects of technology on cesareans, and caution should be exercised when considering technologies. Just as obstetricians are likely to claim great benefits from technology, it is tempting for opponents of technology to attribute all sorts of consequences to its use. In four controlled studies on efficacy of, for example, electronic fetal monitoring (EFM), three found no difference in fetal outcome but did find an increase in sections in the monitored group.[75-77] One study found a benefit and an increase in sections, but the methodology was so problematical as to make the data extremely doubtful.[85] The effect of EFM on cesarean section is extensively discussed in this monograph by Haverkamp and Orleans.

Birth Weight

The fact that babies are getting bigger was frequently cited as a reason for the rising cesarean section rate. This does not appear to be nationally true as the average birth weight has increased barely 2 ounces during the years in which the cesarean rate has doubled.[82] Use of cesarean for very low birth weight babies, however, has increased, and infants now delivered surgically who weigh 1,000 to 1,500 grams are not uncommon.

TABLE II

Deliveries With and Without Complications
United States 1971 - 1980

Year	Number of Deliveries (000)	No Complications (000)	Complications (000)	% Complications
1971	3337	2,771	566	17.0
1972	3224	2,625	599	18.6
1973	3093	2,457	636	20.6
1974	3122	2,392	730	23.4
1975	3048	2,345	703	23.1
1976	3126	2,302	824	26.4
1977	3331	2,390	941	28.2
1978	3361	2,319	1,042	31.0
*1979	3646	1,785	1,861	51.0
1980	3762	1,841	1,921	51.0

Based on data from National Center for Health Statistics; National Hospital Discharge Survey, 1971-1980, Washington, D.C., 1982.

*From 1979 on a coding change caused all multiple births to be listed as complications.

Adapted from Marieskind, H.I. An Evaluation of Caesarean Section in The United States. Washington D.C., Department of Health, Education and Welfare, Office of the Assistant Secretary for Planning and Evaluation/ Health, June, 1979.

Women with Severe Medical Conditions

The tenth factor in the rising rate is due to the medical management of women with severe medical conditions such as diabetes, lupus, or chronic hypertension, enabling many of these women to give birth. Part of their medical management includes delivery by cesarean section.

Herpes II

Herpes II is increasing in the United States and is the eleventh factor contributing to the cesarean rate increase. Nationally, the prevalence of herpes II antibody is estimated at 8% to 12% of the sexually active population, although estimates of the prevalence of herpes II may range from 20% to 50% depending on demographic and socioeconomic characteristics of a given sexually active population. The number of women who come to term with active cervical herpes is estimated to be from 0.5% to 1.5%. Infants infected by herpes II can suffer from brain, kidney, or lung damage or can die. To avoid this possibility, which affects about 85% of newborns born of mothers with active herpes, the child is delivered by cesarean section.[86,87]

Miscellaneous Factors

Other causes of the increase in the rate may depend on individual philosophies; for example, one institution listed multiple pregnancy as an indication for cesarean section. Some physicians advocate cesarean delivery for multiple pregnancies because the second twin is frequently in breech or transverse position. Cesarean delivery is definitely indicated for interlocking twins, but the incidence of this is extremely rare.

Natural childbirth classes have been cited as a reason for the increasing rate. Physicians indicated that many women are unprepared for the realities of labor, believing that breathing and coaching are sufficient. When they go into labor, they are unable to relax and dilatation stops. A cesarean is then needed for delivery. However, one study showed fewer cesarean sections in prepared patients,[88] whereas another showed no difference.[89]

Educational Activities for Expectant Parents

Over the past 5 years numerous classes have been developed to educate parents in childbirth, parenting, and family relationships, and to help them make educated choices regarding childbirth. Courses have also been developed specifically to aid parents whose child will be born by cesarean.[90] Extensive literature is now available on having a positive cesarean experience[7] and on how to avoid unnecessary cesareans.[91]

The need for this preparation is apparent when studies of parent guilt, anger, and disappointment at a cesarean delivery demonstrate the crippling effect the experience can have on bonding and effective parenting.[41]

Cesarean section is a highly useful and essential part of modern obstetrical practice. The extent of its application and its benefits, however, should have been carefully evaluated and scientifically analyzed before it was widely adopted.

It should not be necessary to come later and assess the merits and consequences of a practice when it is already widespread, entrenched, and affecting over 600,000 women and babies every year.

REFERENCES

1. Lowe JA, et al. Caesarean sections in U.S. PAS hospitals. *PAS Rep* 14:1-55, 1976.

2. Hanson H. Revival of the extraperitoneal cesarean section. *Am J Obstet Gynecol* 130:102-103, 1978.

3. Perkins RP. The merits of extraperitoneal cesarean section: A continuing experience. *J Reprod Med* 19:154-158, 1977.

4. Young JH. *Caesarean Section: The history and development of the operation from the earliest times.* London, HK Lewis & Co., 1944.

5. Findley P. *Priests of Lucina: The story of obstetrics.* Boston, Little, Brown & Co, 1939.

6. Cianfrani T. *A short history of obstetrics and gynecology.* Springfield, IL, Charles C Thomas, Publisher, 1960.

7. Donovan B. *The cesarean birth experience.* Boston, Beacon Press, 1977.

8. Duffy J. *The healers.* New York, McGraw-Hill Book Co., 1976.

9. Wertz RC, Wertz DC. *Lying-in: A history of childbirth in America.* New York, The Free Press, 1977.

10. Maxwell AF. Review of 25 years experience in California. *West J Surg* 42:14, 1934.

11. Plass ED, Alvis HJ. A statistical study of 129,539 births in Iowa. *Am J Obstet Gynecol* 28:293-305, 1934.

12. *Health United States, 1980.* Washington, DC, US Government Printing Office, 1980.

13. Placek PJ, Taffel SM. Trends in cesarean section rates for the United States, 1970-78. *Pub Health Rep* 95:540-548, 1980.

14. Shapiro S, et al. *Infant, perinatal, maternal and childhood mortality in the United States.* Cambridge, MA, Harvard University Press, 1968.

15. Pritchard JA, MacDonald PC. *Williams Obstetrics.* (16th ed) New York, Appleton-Century-Crofts, 1980.

16. Burometto E. Trends in cesarean section. *Vital statistics review.* New York State Department of Health, Jan-Mar, 1974.

17. Petitti D, et al. Cesarean section in California—1960 through 1975. *Am J Obstet Gynecol* 133:391-397, 1979.

18. Erhardt C, Gold E. Cesarean section in New York City: Incidence and mortality during 1954-1955. *Obstet Gynecol* 11:241-260, 1958.

19. Butler NR, Alberman E (eds). *Perinatal problems. The second report of the 1958 British Perinatal Mortality Survey.* London, E.S. Livingstone, Ltd., 1969.

20. Placek PJ. *Type of delivery associated with social and demographic, maternal health, infant health and health insurance factors: Findings from the 1972 U.S. National Natality Survey.* Paper presented at the American Statistical Association Meetings, Chicago, Aug 15-18, 1977.

21. Van Praagh I, Tovell H. Cesarean section for fetal distress. *Obstet Gynecol* 31:674-681, 1968.

22. Niswander KR, Gordon M. *The women and their pregnancies. The collaborative perinatal study of the National Institute of Neurological Diseases and Stroke.* Philadelphia, WB Saunders Co., 1972.

23. Klein MD, et al. Primary cesarean section in the multipara. *Am J Obstet Gynecol* 87:242-250, 1963.

24. Gibbons LK: *Analysis of the rise in C-sections in Baltimore.* Doctoral dissertation, Baltimore, School of Hygiene and Public Health, The John Hopkins University, 1976.

25. Johnell HE. Cesarean section: a ten year study. *Acta Obstet Gynecol Scand* 51:231-236, 1972.

26. Ranney B, Stanage WF. Advantages of local anesthesia for cesarean section. *Obstet Gynecol* 45:163-167, 1975.

27. Ranney B, Stanage WF. II. The advantages of local anesthesia for cesarean section (prenatal, neonatal, developmental comparisons, *South Dak J Med* 28:23–31, 1975.

28. *PSRO Hospital Discharge Data Sets*, Jan–Dec 1977. HCFA, Washington, DC, US Government Printing Office, 1978–1979.

29. Department of Health and Social Security: *Report on confidential inquiries into maternal deaths in England and Wales*, 1970–1972. London, Report on Health and Social Subjects, No. 11, 1975.

30. Evrard JR, Gold EM. Cesarean section and maternal mortality in Rhode Island: Incidence and risk factors 1965–1975. *Obstet Gynecol* 50:594–597, 1977.

31. National Institute of Child Health and Human Development (NICHD), Consensus Development Conference on Cesarean Childbirth. *Draft report of the Task Force on Cesarean Childbirth*, Bethesda, MD, National Institutes of Health, 1980.

32. Gibbs RS, et al. The effect of internal fetal monitoring on maternal infection following caesarean section. *Obstet Gynecol* 48:653–658, 1976.

33. Hagen D. Maternal febrile morbidity associated with fetal monitoring and cesarean section. *Obstet Gynecol* 46:260–262, 1975.

34. Shearer M. Complications of cesarean to mother and infant. *Birth Fam J* 4:103–105, 1977.

35. Kuah KB. Labor and delivery after cesarean section. *Aust NZ J Obstet Gynecol* 10:145, 1970.

36. Kuah KB. Delivery after cesarean section. *Br Med J* 3:5, 1969.

37. Morewood GA, et al. Vaginal delivery after cesarean section. *Obstet Gynecol* 42:589–595, 1973.

38. Dewhurst CJ. The ruptured cesarean section scar. *J Obstet Gynaecol Br Emp* 64:113–118, 1957.

39. McGarry JA. The management of patients previously delivered by caesarean section. *J Obstet Gynaecol Br Commonw* 76:137–143, 1969.

40. Shy KK, Logerfo JP, Karp LE. Evaluation of elective repeat cesarean section as a standard of care; application of decision analysis. *Am J Obstet Gynecol* 139:123–129, 1981.

41. Affonso D, Stichler J. Exploratory study of women's reactions to having a cesarean birth. *Birth Fam J* 5:88–94, 1978.

42. Hibbard LT. Changing trends in cesarean section. *Am J Obstet Gynecol* 125:798–804, 1976.

43. Jewett JF. Post-cesarean sepsis. *N Engl J Med* 291:1032–1033, 1974.

44. Ross JE, Galliford BW. Late hemorrhage following cesarean section. *Am J Obstet Gynecol* 119:858–859, 1974.

45. Polishuk WZ, et al. Puerperal endometritis and intrauterine adhesions. *Int Surg* 60:418–420, 1975.

46. Frankel T, Buchsbaum HJ. Vesicocorporeal fistula with menourea. *J Urol* 106:860–861, 1971.

47. Jain SP. Utero-abdominal sinus after classical cesarean section. *J Obstet Gynaecol Br Commonw* 81:333–334, 1974.

48. Schrinsky DC, Benson RC. Rupture of the pregnant uterus: A review. *Ob Gyn Surv* 33:217–232, 1978.

49. Helmkamp BF. Abdominal wound dehiscence. *Am J Obstet Gynecol* 128:803–807, 1977.

50. Arthure H. Maternal deaths from pulmonary embolism. *J Obstet Gynaecol Br Commonw* 75:1309–1312, 1968.

51. Baggish MS, Hooper S. Aspiration as a cause of maternal death. *Obstet Gynecol* 43:327–336, 1974.

52. Crawford JS. The anesthetist's contribution to maternal mortality. *Br J Anaesth* 42:70–73, 1970.

53. Gogoi MP. Maternal mortality from caesarean section in infected cases. *J Obstet Gynaecol Br Commonw* 78:373–376, 1971.

54. Chalmers I, Richards M. Intervention and causal inference in obstetric practice. In *Benefits and hazards of the new obstetrics*, Chard T, Richards M (eds). Philadelphia, JB Lippincott Co, 1977.

55. Maisels MJ, et al. Elective delivery of the term fetus: an obstetrical hazard. *JAMA* 238:2036–2039, 1977.

56. Gluck L, et al. Diagnosis of the respiratory distress syndrome by amniocentesis. *Am J Obstet Gynecol* 109:440–445, 1971.

57. Goldenberg RL, Nelson K. Iatrogenic respiratory distress syndrome. *Am J Obstet Gynecol* 123:617–620, 1975.

58. Hack M, et al. Neonatal respiratory distress following elective delivery: A preventable disease? *Am J Obstet Gynecol* 126:43–47, 1976.

59. Editorial. Cesarean section and respiratory distress syndrome. *Br Med J* 978–979, 1976.

60. Clements JA, et al. Assessment of the risk of the respiratory distress syndrome by a rapid test for surfactant in amniotic fluid. *N Engl J Med* 286:1077–1081, 1972.

61. Lee BO, et al. Ultrasonic determination of fetal maturity at repeat cesarean section. *Obstet Gynecol* 38:294–297, 1971.

62. Lowe JA. Commission on Professional and Hospital Activities, Ann Arbor, MI. Personal communication, May 1978.

63. Marieskind HI. *An Evaluation of cesarean section in the United States*, Washington, DC, US Department of Health, Education and Welfare, 1979.

64. Merrill BS, Gibbs CE. Planned vaginal delivery following cesarean section. *Obstet Gynecol* 52:50–52, 1968.

65. Cragin EB. Conservatism in obstetrics. *NY J Med* 104:1–3, 1916.

66. The American College of Obstetricians and Gynecologists. *Guidelines for vaginal delivery after cesarean childbirth*, ACOG Committee Statement, Jan 7, 1982.

67. Bampton BA, Mancini JM. The caesarean section patient is a new mother too. *JOGN Nurs* 24:58–61, 1973.

68. Jones OH. Cesarean section in present day obstetrics. *Am J Obstet Gynecol* 126:521–530, 1976.

69. National Association for Insurance Commissioners. *Malpractice claims (closed claims study)*. Vol. 4. Milwaulkee, 1977.

70. Murphy H. Delivery following caesarean section—ten years experience at the Rotunda Hospital, Dublin. *J Irish Med Assoc* 69:533–534, 1976.

71. Scully D. *Men who control women's health*. Boston, Houghton Mifflin Co, 1980.

72. Fleck A. Director, Division of Child Health, NY State Department of Health. Personal communication, Nov, 1979.

73. Ott WJ, Ostapowicz F, Meurer J. Analysis of variables affecting perinatal mortality. St Louis City Hospital, 1969–1975. *Obstet Gynecol* 49:481–485, 1977.

74. Eisner V, et al. Improvement in infant and perinatal mortality in the United States, 1965–1973: I. Priorities for intervention. *Am J Public Health* 68:359–366, 1978.

75. Haverkamp AD, et al. The evaluation of continuous fetal heart rate monitoring in high-risk pregnancy. *Am J Obstet Gynecol* 125:310–320, 1976.

76. Haverkamp AD, et al. A controlled trial of the differential effects of intrapartum monitoring. *Am J Obstet Gynecol* 134:399–412, 1979.

77. Kelso IM, et al. An assessment of continuous fetal heart rate monitoring in labor—a randomized trial. *Am J Obstet Gynecol* 131:526–532, 1978.

78. Centers for Disease Control. Reported morbidity and mortality in the United States, 1976. *Morbid Mortal Weekly Rep* 25:1–70, Aug 1977.

79. Haddad H, Lundy LE. Changing indications for caesarean section: A 38-year experience at a community hospital. *Obstet Gynecol* 51:133–137, 1978.

80. Werner EE, et al. *The children of Kanai. A longitudinal study from the prenatal period to age ten.* Honolulu, University of Hawaii Press, 1971.

81. Collea JV, et al. The randomized management of term frank breech presentation: Vaginal delivery vs Caesarean section. *Am J Obstet Gynecol* 131:186–195, 1978.

82. National Center for Health Statistics. *Final natality statistics* 1966–1980. Washington DC, US Government Printing Office, 1981.

83. Miller CA. *What technology breeds—a review of recent U.S. experience with cesarean sections.* The John Sundwall Memorial, School of Public Health, University of Michigan, Ann Arbor, MI, Mar 20, 1978.

84. Thorndike N. *1975 net incomes and work patterns of physicians in 5 medical specialties. Research and statistics note 13.* Health Care Financing Administration, U.S., DHEW, Office of Research and Statistics, July 21, 1977.

85. Renou P, et al. Controlled trial of fetal intensive care. *Am J Obstet Gynecol* 126:470–476, 1976.

86. Corey L. Head of virology, University of Washington, Seattle. Personal communication, July, 1978.

87. Florman AC, et al. Intrauterine infection with *Herpes simplex* virus: Resultant congenital malformations. *JAMA* 225:129–132, 1973.

88. Hughey MJ, et al. Maternal and fetal outcome of Lamaze-prepared patients. *Obstet Gynecol* 51:643–647, 1978.

89. Charles AG, et al. Obstetric and psychological effects of psychoprophylactic preparation for childbirth. *Am J Obstet Gynecol* 131:44–52, 1978.

90. Conner BS, et al. *Manual for setting up prepared childbirth classes for cesarean parents.* Boston, C/SEC Inc, 1976.

91. Young D, Mahan C. *Unnecessary cesareans: Ways to avoid them.* Minneapolis, International Childbirth Education Association, 1981.

SUBMITTED & ACCEPTED: AUGUST, 1982

INDEX